The **Peace Diet**™

Dr. Terry Shintani, M.D., J.D., M.P.H.

The Peace Diet™

Reverse Obesity, Aging and Disease by Eating for Peace of Body, Mind, and Spirit

Terry Shintani, M.D., J.D., M.P.H.

Health Foundation Press

For information contact:
Health Foundation Press
50 S. Beretania St. C-119B
Honolulu, HI 96813

Originally Published in the United States of America
The Peace Diet™ Terry Shintani, M.D., J.D., M.P.H.
10 9 8 7 6 5 4 3 2 1

Layout: Lanilane Ocbina
Cover: Gershom Callada

READ THIS

Before Changing Your Diet

If you have any health conditions or are on medication, you should check with your physician first before starting this diet. Be aware that strict adherence to this diet may require an adjustment in blood sugar and blood pressure medication with the help of your physician in as little as one day. Despite the description of the improvement of health of the many people described in this book and the positive impact this diet may have on various health conditions, the "Peace Diet" is not intended as treatment for any specific disease.

The Peace Diet™

Contents

The Peace Diet™

DEDICATION

To the Almighty Father, the Great Physician, His Son, the Prince of Peace, and all the messengers of peace He has sent to this Earth including YOU.

The Peace Diet™

ACKNOWLEDGEMENTS

There are so many people to thank in producing this book as it has taken a lifetime of my medical training and practice to have the background to write it. I first want to say thanks to my recently departed mentor, Kenneth Francis Brown, with whom I shared a vision of health and peace. He helped me start the non-profit foundation, the Hawaii Health Foundation, where all royalties from this book will go. I want to thank my board members who have supported our work for years including Dr. Earl Bakken, inventor of the wearable pacemaker and founder of Medtronic, (the largest medical device company in the world), Hooipo DeCambra a Robert Wood Johnson Leadership awardee, Jim Jacoby, one of the nation's leading environmentally conscious land developer. My hanai mother Dr. Agnes Cope, my hanai brother, Kamaki Kanahele, Al Harrington (of Hawaii 5-0 fame) and my attorney and law school classmate and friend, Ronald Sakamoto.

I also want to thank Dr. T. Colin Campbell, principal investigator of the China Diet Study, one of the greatest nutrition researchers, who is another mentor of mine. His work has developed much of the science that supports the healthfulness of a plant-based diet. Thanks also goes to Michio Kushi, the founder of the American Macrobiotic movement, who taught me the connection between diet and spirit when I first met him in the 1970's. I also want to acknowledge my friend, Keith Tamura, who introduced me to Macrobiotics when he turned his asthma around with a change in diet.

Thanks also goes to Dr. John McDougall, a true pioneer in plant-based diets for the reversal of disease, who turned his Hawaii practice over to me when he left for California. He was putting science to this concept in the '70's – long before some of the currently well-known proponents of a plant-based diet. I also owe a debt of gratitude to Dr. Walter Willett, my nutrition professor at Harvard University who is now Chief of Nutrition, and along with Dr. Campbell, is one of the greatest nutrition researchers in the world. I also want to acknowledge another one of my Harvard professors, Dr. William Castelli, principal investigator of the Framingham Study, arguably the greatest study on nutrition and heart disease. I am ever grateful for Dr. Claire Hughes, the first Native Hawaiian registered dietitian and co-author of some of my early writings, Dr. Kekuni Blaisdell, my teacher and professor of medicine, and Helen Kanawaliwali O'Connor, a Native Hawaiian healer who was always my partner on our Hawaiian Health projects. Thanks also goes to Dr. Rosanne Harrigan, Chair of the Department of Complementary and Alternative Medicine, who keeps our important work at the University of Hawaii Medical School of Medicine moving forward.

I also have the highest regard for Dr. Keith Block, author of "Life Over Cancer" and founder of the Block Center for Integrative Cancer Therapy; and also Dr. Michael Gregor, whose website www.nutritionfacts.org may be the best nutrition science website on the planet. I consulted them both on a number of nutrition and health issues.

My spiritual teachers have been equally important in the development of this book. While I am Christian and the Prior of the Priory of Hawaii of the Knights of the Orthodox Order of St. John Russian Grand Priory, I owe much gratitude to my parents, Robert and Emi, who taught me both Christian and Buddhist values. I also must thank my adoptive Hawaiian mother, Dr. Agnes Cope, the Chair of the Elders Council of the traditional Hawaiian healers, and my adoptive brother, Kahu Kamaki

xiv

Kanahele, Director of the Native Hawaiian Healing Center, who taught me principles of Hawaiian spiritual healing. He has done prayers with the Dalai Lama and Mother Theresa while working in Washington D.C.

I must also acknowledge the profound influence of the late Dr. Mits Aoki (nicknamed "the Cosmic Dancer") on my understanding of life, death and spirit. He was my Religion professor and often taught in my spiritual development programs. I am also grateful to Countess Nicholas Bobrinskoy, the Grande Dame and Chancellor of the Knights of the Orthodox Order of St. John Russian Grand Priory, who is the great proponent of the continuation of the nearly 1000-year tradition of service of the Hospitallers of St. John, and also Dame Commander, Dr. Sandra Rose Michael, who initiated the creation of Prior of Hawaii and who is the creator of the EES scalar energy generator. I must also acknowledge QiGong GrandMaster, Dr. Effie Chow, for her wisdom that has helped me to understand much about energy medicine.

I also want to acknowledge the spiritual influence and universal teachings of Dr. Jerry Jampolsky, and Dr. Diane Cirincione-Jampolsky, founders of Attitudinal Healing and the use of the 12 Principles of Attitudinal Healing in this book. Thanks also goes to Dr. Diane Nomura, Administrator of the Hawaii Health Foundation and the long time co-host of our radio show, "Healing And You" (which can be heard on AM 1080 in Honolulu or on http://www.kwai1080am.com/ on Sundays at 8pm HST) for many years of helping me keep the Hawaii Health Foundation and our programs on track and for always insisting on including prayer in our programs. She is the author of the book "What the Health" (www.Lulu.com). I would also like to thank Pastor Jeffrey Yamashita, my baptismal pastor for his spiritual support.

Special appreciation goes to Dr. Patricia Bragg, a true "health crusader" who carries on the legacy of the legendary Dr. Paul Bragg, through the Bragg Live Food Products company, and the Director of the company, Dr. John Westerdahl, who have been inspirations in the field of health. They have been consistent sponsors of my radio show along with Down To Earth health food stores who has generously helped my Foundation to put on my "Reverse Disease in 10 Days" Programs. I also want to express my appreciation for my chefs who cooked for my 10 Day health Programs. I consider them my "kitchen pharmacists" including Leslie Ashburn, OriAnn Li, Kathy Maddux, Alyssa Moreau, and Steve Nochese.

I also need to express my appreciation for the Mokichi Okada Association who allows me to use space at their beautiful Wellness Center in Hawaii to house the clinic of the Department of Complementary and Alternative Medicine of the University of Hawaii Medical School. I also appreciate Dr. Raj Kumar, clinical psychologist and meditation teacher and the Gandhi International Institute of Peace for trusting me to be the Chair of their Advisory Board. I don't have permission or space to name the many generous volunteers individually who have blessed our project with their time and effort. They have helped with so many aspects of our work from photography, to cooking, serving food, assisting with set-up, Internet activities and much more, that make our Foundation viable with the modest funds that we have.

I want to thank Pastora Lanilane Ocbina for doing the layout and her associate Gershom Callada, who put together the beautiful graphics in this book. I also want to thank the editor of my book, Dr. Diane Chesson, who is a consummate professional in her work.

Thanks also goes to my family, my brother, Arthur, his wife, Yuko who run our Integrative Wellness Center. Special thanks my wife, Stephanie, and my children, Tracie and Nickie who have put up with me, helped me, and been the source of my strength over the years. Most of all, I thank the Lord for all of these people and the blessings I have been so fortunate to enjoy in my life and for the underlying truths found in this book.

The Peace Diet™

FOREWORD
by Dr. T. Colin Campbell
Professor Emeritus, Cornell University
and author of the "China Study" and "Whole"

I met Dr. Shintani in the early 1990's at an international conference called "Food Choices 2000". One of the first things I noticed about him was that he was a unique medical doctor who had a degree in nutrition from Harvard University. At that conference, I learned about his work with the traditional Hawaiian diet. He worked with arguably one of the most challenging populations with high rates of obesity, diabetes, cancer, and heart disease. He demonstrated that with a change in diet, these diseases could be reversed.

What I thought was intriguing was that the diet that he recommended was fully in line with what I found in the China Diet Study that I had conducted with my colleagues at Oxford and University of Beijing. He used a diet that was low in animal products, low in processed food, and low in fat. Despite the fact that it was high in carbohydrates, he demonstrated that this kind of diet could induce weight loss and improved control of blood sugar, cholesterol and blood sugar.

Because of his findings and his academic background in medicine and nutrition, I invited him to be a visiting professor for one of my classes at Cornell University. It was important for students to hear about Dr. Shintani's work and his finding that a change in diet could induce health improvement that could rival the benefits of prescription medication.

This book describes a dietary approach that I think is excellent for preventing and even reversing a number of diseases. It is certainly good for weight control as he has demonstrated in his peer-reviewed publications. He also describes an approach to nutrition in dealing with whole foods rather than single nutrients that is consistent with some of the concepts in my more recent book, "Whole."

I find Dr. Shintani's work to be very impressive and certainly founded on excellent scientific principles. He actually takes people who are overweight and takes people who have diabetes for example, and he reverses it. He makes people better. The proof is in the pudding.

T. Colin Campbell
Professor Emeritus, Cornell University

PREFACE

I have been conducting health programs for over 25 years now and consistently get people to lose excess pounds, get healthy enough to get off at least some of their medication, and sometimes find inner peace. I've had the good fortune to be able to combine my nutrition background with my practice as a medical doctor along with principles that I learned from my spiritual teachers.

In the early 1990's the U.S. Secretary of Health and Human Services, Donna Shalala gave my health program a national award. It was for the effectiveness of my whole-person health program that included diet, lifestyle, and spiritual principles in a high health-risk Native Hawaiian community. With the results of the program, I demonstrated that by returning an unhealthy population to a traditional diet and lifestyle, their obesity, diabetes, high blood pressure, and other health ailments could easily be remedied.

I hoped that with the added reputation and notoriety that came with such a prestigious award, I might be able to reach many people with a message of health. I have done some of that, especially in Hawaii and the Native Hawaiian community where they arguably have more health problems than any other American sub-group as a result of poverty and obesity-related disease. My health books have reached around the world - some of them translated into Spanish, Japanese, and Chinese, and I have been featured in the Encyclopedia Britannica because of the promising results of my program. Ultimately, however, I would like to take it a step further and help people reach their health and spiritual aspirations as well through the practice of the diet and lifestyle described in this book. Through my experience, I have found that the best diet is one that helps you find inner peace - and then weight control and health follow naturally. When people find themselves on a diet that helps them calm their spirit - the way many people of wisdom have done over millennia, - excess pounds melt away and their health returns. After all, if your spirit is not healthy, then your body and mind are not totally healthy either. And if you nurture the total health of your spirit, then body and mind will follow.

You are the reason this book was written. It is my hope that it will inform and inspire you to choose the path to health, success, happiness and peace, and that through you, others will be informed and inspired. In doing so, I hope to contribute to the movement promoting world health and world peace, one person, one spirit at a time.

Just about every person can heal with the proper diet based on the "Peace Plate," with the eight practices described in this book – and with the help of the Almighty. When healthy in body, mind and spirit, a person can do great things. And when we work together with a healthy spirit, we can heal the world. As the great Mahatma Gandhi once said, "*Be the change you want to see.*"

My Father Had Cancer

Since childhood, I have been aware of the spiritual side of life. I learned to pray when I was very young. When I was 6 months old in 1951, my father was diagnosed with colon cancer. They took out the whole left side of his colon and left him with a permanent colostomy. They said he would be lucky to live another couple of years. My father had a second surgery when I was just 3 years old, and I remember feeling afraid of losing him. Imagine what it's like for a 3-year-old to understand the meaning of the word "metastasis" (the spreading of cancer)? So I began to pray - every night. *"Dear God. Please don't let Dad die of cancer. . ."*

Every single night I prayed that simple prayer - for years - decades. Fortunately, he lived another 40 years and never died of cancer. I will always believe that my prayers had something to do with his survival. After all, how many people do you know of who survived colon cancer in the 1950's? Little did I know then that my Dad having had cancer ultimately, decades later, would lead to my finding a connection between diet, health and peace, and to dedicating my career to helping enhance the lives of as many people as I can.

From Cancer to Peace

Because of this experience, from a young age, I wanted to explore better ways to deal with cancer than what was offered conventionally. After all, doctors didn't seem to have any good answers for my father, and my uncle, who later developed colon cancer and died several months after his diagnosis. I looked into Oriental Medicine, Ayurvedic Medicine, the Gerson Diet, and even Laetrile, purportedly an anticancer substance found in apricot pits.

I first heard about the concept of diet as a path to world peace when I was looking for alternative approaches to dealing with cancer. When I got into law school, I struggled to keep up because I was tired all the time. A friend of mine suggested I try looking into macrobiotics to improve my health and increase my energy. Macrobiotics is primarily known for its dietary approach to health and cancer. It is a whole system of diet and lifestyle that is based on balancing the energies of yin and yang. My friend said that it may help me with my school work. He said that it helped him get rid of his allergies, and his energy and mental alertness improved. Desperate, I tried it. I started eating according to its dietary guidelines. It worked better than I ever expected. My energy returned, and my mind cleared up. My mood and my grades improved. I was determined to learn more about it.

As I began to explore macrobiotics, I was intrigued to learn of many reported cases of people who had reversed cancer, heart disease, diabetes and other diseases using macrobiotics. Interestingly, "One peaceful world" is one of their mottos, and there is a book by that title published by my teacher, Michio Kushi. This puzzled me at first because it seemed strange to talk about world peace in the teachings of healing.

My teacher, Michio Kushi, the father of the American Macrobiotic movement, was in his youth a brilliant political science scholar who studied world government at Tokyo University and Columbia University. Because he witnessed the horrors of World War II and the deaths of many of his close friends in the fire-bombings of Tokyo, his passion was to create a movement to end the need for war. So he diligently studied world government at two of the best universities in the world.

Everything changed when he met George Ohsawa, the founder of macrobiotics. Ohsawa told Kushi that he was a fool if he thought studying world government could lead ultimately to world peace. If the people are unhealthy in body, mind, and spirit, explained Ohsawa, the government will be corrupt no matter how good the governmental system may be. Conversely, if the people are healthy in body mind and spirit, then the government would be healthy, spiritually guided, and world peace would be possible. Ohsawa encouraged Kushi to promote the macrobiotic diet as the pathway to the health of body, mind, and spirit.

I too made this mission my life's path and, in addition to formal training in nutrition at Harvard University after medical school, I have also been formally trained in macrobiotics and the principles of Oriental Medicine at the Kushi Institute and trained in traditional Hawaiian healing by my adopted native Hawaiian family. Remarkably, if you dig deeply enough, you will find that these divergent approaches arrive at the same fundamental truth. You will find that they all acknowledge that the best approach to health is a holistic approach to health including body, mind and spirit, and that the best diet for health and spiritual development is based on whole, unprocessed plant-based food.

Many Have Connected Diet and Peace

My first exposure to how diet affects one's spirit was in experiencing the food served at Buddhist funerals. I grew up in a mixed Christian and Buddhist family, and I noticed that after Buddhist funerals, they would always serve vegetarian food. It was called "shojin ryori" or spiritual development meals. The Buddhist masters believed that plant-based food nurtured the spirit, and that animal-based food would bind your spirit to the earth and make it difficult to spiritually support the departed spirit. For similar reasons "jai," also called "monks' food" in Chinese Buddhist tradition, is vegetarian.

To my surprise, few mainstream experts – scientists, theologians, philosophers, doctors alike – ever talked about the relationship between food and spiritual development. Yet there it was in the Bible and, when I looked further, in the practices of many religions and cultures. Despite differences in belief and practice between Christians and Buddhists, both religions revered plant-based foods.

In the Bible, Genesis 1:29 states that the original God-given diet was plant-based where it says the food includes *"every plant bearing seed . . . and every tree with seed in its fruit . . ."* for humans to eat. In the book of Daniel, Daniel insisted on eating "vegetables" instead of the "king's meat" and he was found to be healthier and better than the king's other advisors. This appreciation of plant-based food is similar to the Buddhist tradition of "shojin ryori" or "spiritual development food" as described above, and to the vegetarian tradition of the Hindu faith.

Many Religions Equate Plant-Based Diet & Peace

On further investigation, I found many more sources from various religions all over the world and from great philosophers and teachers describing how a plant-based diet positively influences our mental and spiritual development. I never read anything purporting that a meat-centered diet could do the same. Quite the contrary, sources suggest that animal flesh, when consumed, hinders the peace-loving spirit.

Modern Movement toward Peace & Plant-Based Diet

Some modern authors too describe the same truth about the relationship between diet and spiritual development, and are worthy of notice. Most notably are books by Dr. Gabriel Cousens who wrote *Spiritual Nutrition,* [1] Stephen Rosen who wrote *Food for the Spirit,*[2] Michio Kushi and Alex Jack who wrote One Peaceful World[3], and Will Tuttle who wrote the *World Peace Diet.*[4] Each of these books describes the healthfulness of a plant-based diet and its value in promoting spiritual development and a sense of personal peace.

My Unique Perspective

But I believe I have a unique perspective as a nutritionist, practicing physician, and medical school professor. I am one of relatively few physicians who have credentials in nutrition, have conducted research, and also practice medicine with real patients. I have also been formally trained in what might be called "alternative" health systems such as macrobiotics and traditional Hawaiian healing (the ancient healing arts of Hawaii). I have also engaged in spiritual development training that incorporates diet and lifestyle to improve health. I have personally experienced an elevation of spirit while on a strict "Peace Diet" for spiritual development.

When following the guidelines of the Peace Diet, I have personally experienced an elevation in energy, mood, and awareness. I have had experiences and insights of things to happen in the future that I could not explain otherwise except that the Diet elevated my consciousness, enabling me to tap into some higher consciousness. I have accomplished things in my career that I never thought possible. For example, I credit this higher consciousness that opened me to the guidance of the Almighty with how we were able to create a health program that won a National award with essentially no funding. It was so successful that we were featured in Newsweek, CBS This Morning, CNN news, Dateline NBC and in the Encyclopedia Britannica.

In addition, for over 20 years I have conducted health programs based on a plant-based diet and improved the health of thousands of people who have come through my programs and practice. I have seen individuals lose hundreds of pounds and cholesterol numbers, blood pressures, blood sugars, and countless ailments improve on a plant-based diet based on the concepts I recommend in this book. It has always impressed me that a diet that is good for the spirit is also the best diet for the mind and body.

As with my other books, this book is about nutrition, and yet the focus is a little different from my other books. First, it is a much simplified version of the diet that I recommend. It is certainly about improving our health, losing excess pounds, and feeling better than ever. But it is also about a missing element in nutrition that is often neglected but in many ways may be more important than dealing with weight, diabetes, heart disease, and other chronic ailments. It is about how diet affects our personal peace and even world peace as described by many philosophers and writers before me.

This focus on nutrition leading to peace, coupled with my career-long practice of "lifestyle medicine" and "whole-person" health programs where I experienced not just the medical and health results of a good diet, but also the spiritual effects, as well as my witnessing greater intuition, more lucid dreams, and near psychic effects has led me to write this book. It is my hope that it may help you in your own path to health, enlightenment and peace.

"Behold, I have given you every plant yielding seed which is upon the face of all the earth, and every tree with seed in its fruit; you shall have them for food."
- Genesis 1:29

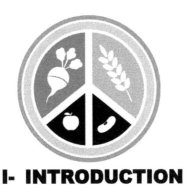

I- INTRODUCTION

The Book You've Been Looking For

This may be the book you have been looking for. The fact that you are reading these words in this book is no accident. Call it synchronicity, coincidence, guidance from the universe or the hand of God; in whatever way you choose to describe it, you are reading this book for a reason that may change your life.

You have been guided to these pages to explore this way of controlling your weight, optimizing your health, reducing your need for medication, and elevating your mood and spirit. In this book I want to share a simple secret of the ages with you. I want to show you how to control your weight, reverse disease, chronic pain, and the aging process by creating peace of body, peace of mind, and peace of spirit.

The Best Diet in the World

I want to introduce you to the best diet in the world. This is not just my opinion. It is the opinion of many people in the field of health, doctors, nutritionists, celebrities, athletes, leaders, and especially great souls throughout history. The principles behind this diet are found in modern health books, ancient holy books, popular books, and scientific journals. This diet allows you to eat as much as you want and still lose weight, while at the same time regaining your health. Many people on this diet have regained energy and reduced or eliminated their need for medication. Here is what one patient says:

> *"I've lost weight - about 50 pounds."* . . . *I was taking 75 units [of insulin] a day and taking four high blood pressure pills. . . But after 10 days, my insulin count went down to 5 units a day and my cholesterol went down to about 100 and I don't need blood pressure medicine anymore."* Ronald N.

This diet, which I call the Peace Diet, has allowed some people to lose over a hundred pounds without counting a single calorie. Many have seen their aches and pains disappear, their headaches gone, and their fatigue and depression evaporate. Other people swear that it has improved their energy and spiritual development.

> *"Somehow, eating this way, my mind is clearer, my consciousness is elevated and my prayers seem more effective."* John W.

Why do I call it the best diet in the world? Well, what other diet allows you lose weight without counting calories or portion size, has been shown to reverse heart disease, diabetes, hypertension and other health problems, is associated with better mood, and has been recommended through the ages for spiritual development? In addition, it helps the environment, reduces the suffering of animals, and reduces karmic debt. It's a diet that produces real results in real people who see their blood sugar, cholesterol, blood pressure, and many other ailments improve. It's a diet that helps people feel better physically, mentally, emotionally, and spiritually.

Not a Fad Diet

The Peace Diet is not a "fad diet." It is not a diet that carries the name of a famous doctor. It does not bear the name of some trendy place or food. It is not named after some catchy principle that has been invented in the last few years. It is not based on one or two nutrients or metabolic process. Instead, it is based on principles that are thousands of years old and validated by modern science. It is based on a few timeless principles that bring into play the full complexity of the interaction of whole food on the whole of human physiology.

The Peace Diet developed out of my own search for health and energy in which I discovered a way of eating that ultimately changed my life. Changes to my eating habits not only caused natural weight loss and improvement in health, but also elevated my mind and my spirit. This has enabled me to find the mental energy to earn four college degrees, and the spiritual guidance to apply this knowledge to help those who need it most. In a nutshell, this is what I have learned since adhering to the Peace Diet in my own life:

> *"Sow a healthy diet, reap a healthy body; sow a healthy body, reap a healthy spirit; sow a healthy spirit, reap a healthy world."*

It is my deep belief that a truly healthy world means a peaceful world, and that peace within a person leads to peace in his/her interactions with others.

Diet for Body, Mind, and Spirit

I have learned that a diet that is healthy for the spirit is going to be the best diet for the mind and body. Think about it. Ask yourself, if your spirit is not healthy, are you ever truly and completely healthy? Ask yourself, if you are taking medication, are you every truly healthy? Is your body ever at peace? Or do the medications fix one problem and cause problems elsewhere? Then ask yourself, what is the best diet and lifestyle that supports the health of your body, mind and spirit?

If you want to know the answer, consider the wisdom of spiritually developed people throughout the ages and couple it to modern science and actual clinical results of people who have tried it. Then, consider trying the Peace Diet because it is a way of life to support the health of your spirit as well and your mind and body. And because it will support the health of spirit, mind and body, it is also the best way to lose weight, get physically healthy, reduce or eliminate the need for medication, and keep you truly healthy in the long run.

Why the Peace Diet?

I call it the Peace Diet because I have found that eating in a way that brings peace and harmony to your bodily processes brings natural weight control, and optimal physical, mental and spiritual health. In other words, I have found that eating in a way that minimizes the metabolic wars going on in your body brings natural weight control and reversal of disease, as well as the elevation of your mind and spirit. My experience and that of others is that if you follow the Peace Diet carefully, you may find yourself feeling less stress, less discomfort, and more energy, calmness, and personal peace as a result.

In the process of gaining peace of body, mind and spirit, you may find pounds falling off and your health returning. It does so because no longer will your body have to fight so many metabolic battles that result in fatigue, overweight and disease. No longer will you have to battle your hunger drive to control your weight. Your body will function the way nature intended it to function. People throughout the ages have used this diet to help them find inner peace. People in modern times can use it to find weight control and health as well.

I also call this the "Peace Diet" because it is based on a diagram that looks like the simple universal "Peace Sign" that describes the diet in a simple, easy-to-use manner as you will see. The fact that people find natural weight loss and improvement in their blood pressure, blood sugar, and cholesterol is probably the best evidence that it is the right kind of diet to follow.

The Peace Diet for Weight Control

The Peace Diet is a proven method for effective weight control. I spent 18 years at a community health center in Hawaii serving an ethnically mixed, largely native Hawaiian population, one of the most obesity-prone populations in the world. I worked in family practice and preventive medicine programs. Some of my patients were 300, 400, 500, even 600 pounds; my largest was 890 pounds. Many were living in poverty, which meant that they tended to eat more convenience food and fast food. Of course, whether we live in poverty or not, processed, convenience-type food greatly increases our risk of obesity.

Perhaps the most obvious and immediate benefit of the Peace Diet, which calls for removing processed foods from one's diet, is weight loss. Margaret, one of my most memorable patients, lost 70 pounds in 6 months. She wound up losing nearly half of her 243 pounds-- and has kept it off for years. This is what Margaret says about being on my health Program:

> *"When I started the program, I weighed 243 pounds. Currently, I weigh about 128 pounds. I'm kinda going in between 125 and 130 pounds. The other thing too is that I thought, now my outside matches my inside. You know, now I look like how I feel on the inside. My cholesterol used to be 223. Now, almost two years after the program, it stays at around 131. I recommend this program to anyone, and if you don't make it complicated, if you follow it, it's really not hard."* Margaret F.

The Peace Diet and Health

As you can see from this participant's example, it isn't just weight that is controlled. Cholesterol is reduced, sometimes as much as 100 points in three weeks. Blood pressure improves, sometimes in as little as one or two days. Blood sugar levels are also positively affected by the Peace Diet, despite the fact that there is no portion-size restriction and it is typically high in carbohydrates.

Another of my patients, who was on 120 units of insulin before she began to follow the Peace Diet, was able to control her blood sugar without taking insulin shots within only ten days. In her words:

> *When I started the program, I was taking 120 units of insulin, and on the 10th day, I had to stop taking insulin altogether because my blood sugars were getting too low. Now, one year later, I've lost around 35 to 40 pounds and I'm still off insulin.* Joanne G

The Peace Diet and Spirit

People following this eating program notice that their energy increases and their mood is better. Here is the comment of another Peace Diet follower:

> *What I found is that with this program, I feel very light, I have a lot of energy.* Arlene R.

> *I feel wonderful. Every day I get up, and I feel happy.* Melissa T.

In addition, some people start noticing inexplicably that their spiritual consciousness increases. This is just what is described in ancient texts and quotes from spiritual teachers. I'll continue to point out again and again that the best diet for health is one that improves the spirit as well as the body and mind.

> *"When one becomes a vegetarian, it purifies the soul"* – Isaac Bashevis Singer, Author, Nobel laureate

> *"A vegetarian diet elevates the spirit and makes meditation much more effective"* Sooriya Kumar, www.mounafarm.org

The Peace Plate

The Peace Plate is how I describe the way the general proportions of food should look on your plate. To picture this, think of the way the peace sign itself looks: a circle divided down the center vertically with dividing lines starting at the center of the vertical line and angling downwards symmetrically on each side, ending at the edge of the circle. Now imagine that there is a peace sign on your dinner plate itself.

Dr. Shintani's
PEACE PLATE

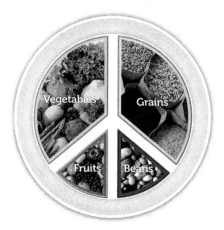

On the left side of the plate, the larger top section covering about 30 to 35% of the plate should be filled with vegetables, with the smaller section at the bottom left reserved for fruit-- about 15% to 20% of the plate. On the right hand side, whole grains should occupy the larger top section, again representing about 30 to 35% of the plate. Beans & legumes round out the lower right space of the Peace Plate configuration, occupying the remaining 15-20% of the circle.

If you follow the guidelines described in this book for constructing the Peace Plate at every meal, a process which also includes using unprocessed food, chewing properly, eating with gratitude, eating foods in season, and eating in harmony with your locality, you will have a diet that supports good health. Your diet will also be a rough modern equivalent to the *"shojin ryori*," or the Zen concept of diet for spiritual development, which is discussed later in this book.

Whole Person Peace Plan Includes 8 Enhancing Factors

This diet doesn't stop with the dinner plate, however. Supporting the Peace Plate are eight enhancements forming the basis of a lifestyle that can improve health and elevate the spirit. The first four are environmental: energy, air, water, and earth. In other words, it is important to optimize your exposure to energy, clean air, pure water, and natural elements of the earth, by which I mean minerals and molecules.

The second four enhancements to the Peace Plate are based on intention: activity, thoughts, love, and prayer. As you read through this book and come to understand all the guidelines of the Peace Diet, from the food you eat to the environment you surround yourself with, to the behavior you employ, you will see that all of it is consistent with the recommendations of both ancient wisdom and modern science.

The Peace Diet is Based on Timeless Principles

The Peace Diet is based on timeless principles that have been taught for millennia by physicians and philosophers alike. Some of the principles may be found in Ayurvedic medicine as well as traditional Chinese medicine. It may be found in Buddhist philosophy as well as the Holy Bible. The effectiveness of these principles of the Peace Diet has also been supported by modern peer-reviewed science.

In the next chapter, I'll describe five basic lessons that will help you to understand some of the universal principles behind the Peace Diet. It will help you realize that food was made a certain way in nature for a reason and that eating food that is altered and out of balance will alter our health.   This will help you to realize that the laws of nature are always working and that everything is connected.   It will help you see that when you have peace at a molecular level, you will lay the foundation for the peace and health of body, mind and spirit.

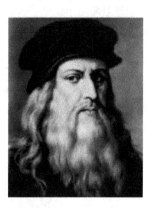

"Truly man is the king of beasts, for his brutality exceeds theirs. We live by the death of others: We are burial places!"
-Leonardo Da Vinci (1452-1519)

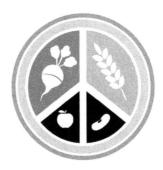

II- FIVE LESSONS FOR WEIGHT CONTROL, HEALTH, AND PEACE

I have been very fortunate to have learned from many of the best teachers in the world academically, spiritually and experientially. Some of my best teachers are my patients and volunteers, and even my wife and daughters have been great teachers to me. I'll never forget that I learned from Dr. Jerry Jampolsky, founder of Attitudinal Healing that everyone is a teacher, and everyone is a student. We should also never forget what we can learn from observing animals and nature and messages we get through the small voice within and the great voice without that we tap into through meditation and prayer.

When I was studying nutrition at Harvard University, I also had the opportunity to study at night an "East-West" approach to healing. It was at the Kushi Institute where they taught Macrobiotics, a system of healing based on understanding of the laws of nature and balancing the forces of yin and yang. Michio Kushi was one of my esteemed teachers. In Kushi's "The Book of Macrobiotics," he makes an important statement that I think all those who seek to heal themselves, all healers, and leaders of the world should take to heart. He says:

> *The Order of the Infinite Universe - the eternal principles of change - are nothing but the different names of the living God or the moving infinite creation. . . Without knowing the Order of the Universe, it is fruitless to talk about life or truth, and it is senseless to speak of*

human existence and life. Without understanding the Order of the Universe, no one can achieve health, freedom, and happiness through his or her own initiative.[5]

The following five lessons are general lessons that I have learned from my many great teachers about how the universe works in relation to your weight control, health and peace.

Lesson One: Eating for Peace of Body, Peace of Mind and Peace of Spirit Induces Natural Weight Control and Health

I've lost 93 lbs. Losing weight is not going to cure everything, but physically I feel so good. It really has made a difference. I feel wonderful, I have tons of energy.   Melissa T.

I lost 7-1/2 pounds in 10 days. I'm really happy now. With this program, I feel lighter, I feel leaner, I feel happier.
Lynne K.

I've been treating patients, researching, and writing about nutrition for over 25 years, and I've been reading diet books for nearly 40 years. I've seen fad diets come and go. The truth about diets is that they all work, but in general they all fail. Why? There are two main reasons: Imperfect diets and imperfect people.

Any man-made diet which focuses on a single nutrient or a single metabolic concept is bound to have problems. Low-carb, high-carb, high-protein, low-fat, 30-40-30% nutrients, good fat, good carb, gluten-free, grain-free, candida, immune power, blood type, and so forth, are all single concept diets. These all fail in the end because food -- and its effect on our physiology -- is too complex of an interaction to be attached to an individual nutrient or metabolic concept. Dr. T. Colin Campbell, emeritus professor of Cornell University, eloquently makes this point in his book "Whole."

There are, in fact, myriad factors affecting our weight and overall health: Calories, fats, type of fats, hydrogenated fats, carbs, type of carbs, form of the carbs, proteins, types of protein, glycemic index, glycemic load, insulin, insulinemic index, insulin load, the processing of carbs, the processing of food, fiber content, type of fiber, the weight of the food, how much you chew your food, antioxidants, vitamins, minerals, chromium, genes, epigenetics (how food turns on or off various genes), allergens, gliadins, the cooking of food, the type of gut flora, inflammation, grehlin, leptin, cholecystokinin, the stretching of the stomach, stress, hormones, cortisol, thyroid, estrogen, progesterone, growth hormone, testosterone, sleep, exercise, pollutants, GMO foods, xenoestrogens (external estrogen analogs), toxins, pesticides, herbicides, aspartame, infection, balance of energy, balance of nutrients… to name just a few! The futility of dealing with only one or two of these factors should be obvious.

The Peace Diet is based on an appreciation of the fact that there are many battles going on within the body to balance all of the above factors especially when we eat improperly. This Diet is based on the idea that having too many battles going on in your body at the same time can cause weight gain, disease, fatigue, and chronic pain. And conversely, bringing peace to these processes will induce natural weight control and the health of body, mind and spirit.

If we eat in a way that deals with just one dietary factor or one metabolic process in isolation, we may be creating other problems. For example, if we follow a "high protein" diet, we may wind up eating too much protein that can cause acidification of the blood, loss of calcium, and increased inflammation. If we follow a "low fat" diet, we may wind up eating too many processed carbs and increase the risk of diabetes.

The Peace Diet makes optimal use of whole foods and the complex interactions of human physiology and anatomy. It doesn't focus on a single nutrient or metabolic concept, nor does it attempt to be low fat or low carb, because when following the Peace Diet guidelines, your food will naturally be high in fiber, high in bulk, low in fat, and high in unprocessed carbohydrates. There is no need to focus on a specific nutrient or metabolic function. When following Peace Diet guidelines, your food will be naturally rich in vitamins, minerals, antioxidants, and necessary nutrients in the right form and proportions that will minimize your metabolic battles and bring peace to your body, mind and spirit.

We should consider many perspectives

We should also consider many perspectives. For example, some will consider the single concept that we should avoid carbohydrates to restore good health and eliminate problems such as obesity, diabetes disease, and other problems. As a result, the recommendation is to replace the carbohydrates with protein and fat from animal products. However, such an approach ignores the fact that the populations that consume the most carbohydrates have the least amount of obesity and diabetes such as in Japan and China. When they start consuming fewer carbohydrates and more meat and protein, diabetes and obesity rates increase. Looking only at limiting carbohydrates also ignores the fact that carbohydrates behave very differently depending on whether they are whole or processed. The same amount of carbohydrate in the form of whole grain has a very different effect on blood sugar and insulin when compared to carbohydrates in the form of flour products.

In our 10-Day Program, we use what might be considered a high-carbohydrate diet and we still induce natural weight control and reversal of diabetes. Moreover, current science supports the healthfulness of diets that are high in unprocessed grains, vegetables, and fruit, and very low in flesh consumption. In addition, we should take into account the wisdom from many cultures indicating that eating the flesh of dead animals is not healthy for the body, the mind or the spirit.

> *Kill not, neither eat the flesh of your innocent prey, lest you become the slaves of Satan.* Jesus (in the Essene Gospel of Peace, Book 1)

What makes the Peace Diet unique is that it places value on the complex interactions that occur between natural food and the human body, mind and spirit, and seeks to put food on the plate in such a way that those interactions – the ones that will bring peace to our bodily metabolism – will indeed take place. It also takes into account ancient wisdom and modern science. With these healthy connections being made between our food and our bodies, we improve not only our physical health, but our spiritual health as well, a connection reflected in our growing sense of inner peace and joy.

Following a proper diet is one of the ways we achieve what some people call "oneness" with nature and the universe, a principle at the core of the Peace Diet. Much more than simply a food prescription, this diet is about eating and living in such a way that leads us to achieve physical, mental, emotional, and spiritual health, which then leads us to harmony with the world around us by virtue of the fact that our bodies are at peace with food from the Earth in its natural form.

Lesson Two: You Are What You Eat

Your diet affects your physical body and physical health more than any other factor. What you eat can have a profound effect on the shape of your body. In addition, for dealing with most health problems that we face today, a healthy diet is usually more effective than medication. Of course, you also need air and water to live, and other factors influence your health too, but the food you eat literally *becomes* who you are: the molecules in your food eventually become your tissue, bones, muscle and brain.

Virtually all of your body including bone is replaced every few days to every 3 to 7 years depending on the type of tissue. The food literally becomes you, so you can see how the quality of the food you eat will affect the quality of your physical body! There is no doubt about this. Indeed, poor quality food is responsible for most of the chronic diseases suffered in the industrialized world, and is beginning to affect all populations that begin to modernize their food systems. What is happening is that the unnatural and processed food we consume causes our bodies to fight for balance and to fight off harmful foods and the result is weight gain, fatigue, disease and even death.

The Peace Diet can remedy many of these chronic conditions by bringing peace to our metabolism. As mentioned earlier, natural weight control is only the first of a long list of health improvements: Blood sugar, blood pressure, cholesterol, arthritis, allergies, and more. Thus, a common result of the Peace Diet is a reduction in the need for medication in many people who follow it.

> *I have high blood pressure, high cholesterol, and migraine headaches. . . I was taking at least 8 medicines....In 3 days I got off my high blood pressure medicine and on the 4th day I got off my migraine medicine."*   Karen T.

> *My doctor couldn't believe it when I lost 16 pounds in 6 weeks. My blood sugar dropped to 89, so Dr. Shintani took me off my diabetes medicine.* Anne H.

More explanation and examples of specific diseases follow in chapters to follow on health.

Lesson Three: Food Affects Your Mind and Mood

Participants in my program notice a change in mood, confidence, and energy level, and some find a deeper level of spiritual consciousness. This is because there is a definite relationship between what you eat and your level of happiness...or unhappiness. Bringing peace to your body can also bring peace to your mind and mood.

> *Whenever I eat this way, I feel so much better, I don't need as much sleep and I'm more active.* Jerry T,

> *I like how I feel. It's really been wonderful. I have more energy.* Sarah M.

MaryAnn, a petite, trim, healthy-looking woman of less than 5 feet tall weighed about 90 pounds. In spite of a healthy appearance, MaryAnn had very high levels of cholesterol and triglycerides. She did well in the program, and at the end, when I asked people to share their thoughts about the Peace Diet, I was happy to see her raise her hand. I expected to hear the story of how she lowered her cholesterol and triglycerides, but instead, MaryAnn surprised me by telling the group assembled before her that her husband loves the program.

MaryAnn explained that even though her husband was not on the diet, he wanted her to stay on it forever. Since beginning the Peace Diet her husband had noticed that MaryAnn's grouchiness had gone away! Being on the Peace Diet had completely changed her mood.

I've heard countless similar stories of how people who followed these dietary recommendations have also begun to feel better, to have more energy, and to have a generally more positive outlook than they did before changing their diets.

There is such a clear connection between food and mental state that scientists such as Judith Wurtman PhD of MIT have written books such as "Managing Your Mind and Mood Through Food" about how diet can affect mood and mind.

Meat-Eating May Cause People to be Stubborn

From an Eastern medicine perspective of balancing yin and yang, food can have a profound effect on mood and mental state. For example, eating lots of meat can cause people to become rigid in their thinking and stubborn. Meat is a very "yang" food and is contractive rather than expansive. As a result, people become narrow-minded rather than open-minded and judgmental and set in their ways. When I ask heavy meat-eaters if they are willing to give up meat eating, they will typically dig their heels in and refuse.   That is their meat talking - typically making them unwilling to change. This is why it usually takes a disease, pain or some other motivation for meat-eaters to change. The flip side is that when people eat lots of sugar and processed food which is "yin" they become wishy-washy and indecisive.

Using this concept in balancing the diet with whole unprocessed plant-based food helps people to be open minded, adaptive and peaceful according to these ancient principles of yin and yang. For example, the luminary from Japan, Mokichi Okada who founded the Church of the World Messianity and the Mokichi Okada Association pointed out that:

> *When people continue to eat a vegetarian diet, their states of mind are different. Excessive discontent and complaints dwindle away to*

nothing. They do not get angry. . . . These changes are truly remarkable. Distress and hardships disappear to a considerable degree. Their tolerance is excellent.[6]

Rudolf Steiner, founder of the Waldorf Schools and the Anthroposophical Society pointed out the importance of his vegetarian diet in his ability to do enormous amounts of work - mostly mental in nature - in this statement:

> *I myself have known that I would have been unable to go through strenuous activities of the last 24 years without vegetarian nutrition* (Rudolf Steiner, Nutrition and Health: Lectures of the Workmen: Anthroposophical Press, NY, 1987*).*

Lesson Four: Diet and Spirit are Connected

The connection between diet and spiritual health does not have published science behind it because there are no convenient scientific measures of spiritual health. For this lesson, I point out that we must not forget the spiritual side of life despite the fact that it is not measurable. We must acknowledge that science isn't everything - and while it may provide some of the truth about how to manage our health, it is certainly not the whole truth. We have to realize that absence of proof is not proof of absence. I believe that a lot of knowledge comes from scientists and research, but wisdom comes from elders, observation and prayer.

In looking at the videos of the great tsunami of 2004 in Indonesia, a number of observers were puzzled. "Why are there no dead animals?" they wondered.

Bodies of dead humans lay all over the place, but not animals. In a January 4, 2005 article in National Geographic News, it was reported that just before the tsunami struck,

"According to eyewitness accounts, the following events happened:
- Elephants screamed and ran for higher ground.
- Dogs refused to go outdoors.
- Flamingos abandoned their low-lying breeding areas.
- Zoo animals rushed into their shelters and could not be enticed to come back out."

Perhaps, having lived more in harmony with nature, the animals "sixth sense" had been developed, and they sensed that something terrible was going to happen. In response, they headed for the hills before the catastrophe occurred.

In the book of Daniel, an Old Testament story of the Holy Bible, Daniel and his friends consumed a plant-based diet for 10 days. At the end of this time, he and his friends were judged to be healthier-looking and 10 times smarter than those who ate rich food from the King's table. Daniel later was able to save the lives of King Nebuchadnezzar's advisors by giving the King an interpretation of his dreams. Daniel pointed out that he was able to receive the interpretation that came from God. No one can say for certain that his diet helped to open his spiritual connection to God, but who can say that the diet did not help?

Of course, no peer-reviewed research papers exist to validate this premise, but for such spiritual phenomena, there probably never will be. The point is that according to the best evidence available, ancient and modern writings of many wise men and women, a plant-based diet brings you into a closer relationship with the harmony and rhythms of the universe. It affects your spirit, your connection to God, your connection to the universe.

From my own personal experience, I have had many instances of enhanced prayers and even what people might consider pre-cognitive vision. As a Christian, I always attribute this to the answering of my prayers just as was the case when I was a child praying that my father would not die of cancer. I can't help but believe that my change to a plant-based diet and the avoidance of flesh food enhanced my ability to communicate with the almighty Father.

For example, my job with the Native Hawaiian community on the remote side of Oahu came about as a result of prayer. When I saw the high rates of obesity, diabetes, and chronic disease there, I prayed and a vision of the Hawaii Diet program came to me. When I found that there was no funding for such a project, I prayed and the message came back to me in my prayers. The message I received was this.

> *Ask and it shall be given; seek and ye shall find; knock and it shall be opened.*

When I knocked on doors for help with the project, I was trying to create a budget to see how much funding we needed. Instead, so many people offered help, free rental space, food and everything we needed that we did not have to raise additional funds. When the project won a national award, and I presented it at the NIH, we had to declare our funding sources to disclose any potential conflict of interest. You could hear a gasp in the audience when I declared that we were an unfunded project. I will always attribute the success of the projects I have conducted to the hard work of people who were kind enough to work with me and helped us with goods and services and most of all to prayer and the Almighty.

When our project won the national award from the U.S. Secretary of Health and Human Services, a story about our project appeared in Newsweek magazine. Because of the response I received from all around the world, from people interested in being on my Program, my father's friend suggested that I meet

Mr. Kenny Brown who at the time was the Chairman of the Board of Queen's Health Systems, the largest hospital system in Hawaii. He cautioned me, however, not to waste his time and to go in with a plan.

I prayed for hours on this plan. In my prayers, it came to me that because people were calling from all around the world, Hawaii would one day become a world center for health. This made sense because Hawaii had the best water, the cleanest air, and had an ancient healing tradition in its cultural history.

Because of this vision, I "photoshopped" a picture of the world with Hawaii at the center of this picture with arrows coming out from Hawaii showing that health would emanate from Hawaii. Below is the picture that I had prepared.

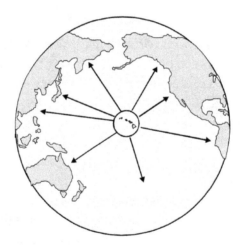

Bear in mind how unusual a diagram this is because Hawaii is never placed at the center of the world in a world map. Anyone who wants such a picture has to do some work cutting, pasting and reshaping in order to get this kind of map.

When I arrived at Mr. Brown's office, he was very warm and complimented me on the work I had done with the Native

Hawaiian community. Then he showed me a flip chart of what was being done at the Queen's Hospital system. In the midst of his presentation, he flipped a chart and the following diagram was one that he had had his people put together.

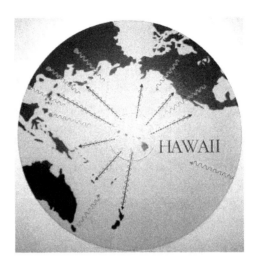

The similarity was striking, as anyone can see. When I saw his diagram, my mind started reeling, and the hair stood up on the back of my neck. I thought to myself, "The Lord has spoken to both of us."

Mr. Brown then turned to me and said, "Well, what do you think of what we're doing?"

I then flipped my presentation to my diagram and I told him, "I don't know how to tell you this, but I came to show you the same thing."

Mr. Brown looked at my diagram, and I could sense his wonderment at the similarity of our diagrams. He then looked at me and said, "Well, I guess we have to do something together, don't we?"

He then arranged for a substantial grant from his organization to start up my Project. We both knew that we had both been in spiritual communication with the Lord, and this was good evidence.

Rudolf Steiner, luminary of the late 1800's and early 1900's, founder of the Anthroposophical Society and the Waldorf Schools was one of Europe's great spiritual teachers in his day. He clearly connected the vegetarian way of eating with an improvement of spiritual health. In one of his lecture in 1909 as translated in a collection of his lectures on nutrition, he said:

> *A time will come when a vegetarian diet will be valued much more highly than is the case today. . . . They will realize then that their whole physical and spiritual horizon can be widened through a vegetarian diet. . . .*

More Than a Road Map to Peace

More than just a dietary road map, the Peace Diet way of eating appears to sharpen your intuition simply by bringing you into a closer relationship to that which sustains you. I go so far as to say that the Peace Diet awakens our sense of spiritual connectivity with the universe and all it does to produce the food we consume and provide us with all the elements for a healthy body, mind and spirit. This connection is, I think, described well in the Bible, when John writes in his gospel:

> *The wind blows wherever it pleases. You hear its sound, but you cannot tell where it comes from or where it is going. So it is with everyone born of the Spirit.* John 3:8

The Peace Diet appears to open the door to an awareness of spirit, improving our ability to be in sync with the workings of the world around us, from the inside out.

Lesson 5: Everything Is Connected

One of the most important lessons of the Peace Diet is that everything is connected. Total health and weight control is not just about food. The Peace Diet is about everything that we consume including food, water, air, energy, thoughts and feelings. It is about being at peace with heaven and earth, physically and spiritually. It is being in an overall harmonious resonance of our outer environment with our inner intentions and actions. Everything is connected - from the molecular to the infinite. I believe that if we are healthy at the molecular level, we will be healthy at our physical level. If we are healthy physically, we will be healthy mentally. If we combine physical health with positive intention mentally, we will be healthy spiritually. And if we are spiritually healthy, we can resonate with the universe and with other spiritually healthy souls. And together, we can have a positive impact on the world.

Of course, if you follow the Peace Diet way of eating, you will lose weight if you are overweight, (100% of the overweight participants in my Programs lose weight) and your health numbers will improve. However, other factors such as exercise, rest, meditation, positive attitude and prayer can all play a role in creating peace of body, peace of mind, peace of spirit, and your overall health.

The connection between mind, body and spirit goes both ways. Peace of body affects peace of mind and spirit. Peace of mind and spirit affects the health of your body. There is a whole field of study called "Psychoneuroimmunology" that researches and documents the connection between mental attitude and how it affects your immune system and your health.

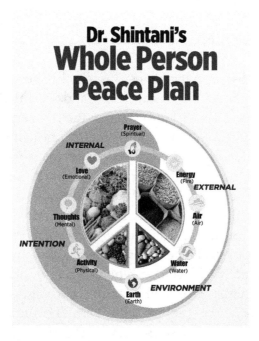

The great Shaolin monks of China follow a plant-based diet and are noted for their legendary strength and physical prowess in the fighting arts. As a testament to the effectiveness of their practices, they have been the seat of Chinese martial arts, kung fu, tai chi and qigong for 1500 years.

It has been said that if you want to explode the myth of needing to eat meat for strength, just say two words, "Shaolin monk." But in order to develop their skill and strength, they engage in other activities beyond just diet. They engage in vigorous exercise and physical training, and they also engage in meditation, prayer and clean positive living.

In a later chapter, I describe four external and four internal factors you should consider to optimize your health in addition to diet. The external factors are represented by earth, air, energy and water. We need to be sure that we are exposed to the right kind and amount of solid substances (food, herbs, supplements, chemicals), clean air, energy (e.g., sunlight, radiation), and clean water. These are important because if we are exposed to a toxic environment, our bodies are constantly doing battle to ward off the effects of these toxins and pollutants. This disrupts our bodily peace and contributes to health problems.

Conversely, proper exposure to and balancing of these factors can greatly influence our health and peace. For example, breathing properly (air) greatly enhances meditation and can alkalize your blood. Balancing the body's energy has been shown to help resolve many health conditions through modalities such as acupuncture, bio-modulation, and scalar energy.

The four internal factors are based on our own intentions. They are exercise, thoughts, love and prayer. These correspond to physical, mental, emotional and spiritual health practices. While I believe that diet is the most important determinant of your health, these other aspects are also important contributors to maintaining bodily peace and your overall health.

These eight factors are represented as eight icons in a circle around the Peace Diet Plate diagram. It is described in detail in chapter X. When you are able to follow the Peace Diet and optimize these eight factors in your life, you bring peace to your body's physiology and you lay the foundation for physical, mental, emotional, and spiritual health. And because everything is connected, you will find that you may influence the health of others, and have the potential for contributing to healing the world.

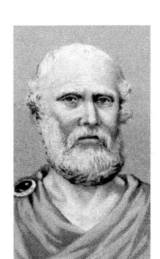

"The gods created certain kinds of
beings to replenish our bodies...
they are the trees and the plants
and the seeds."
-PLATO (circa 428-347 B.C.)

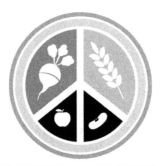

III- EAT MORE, WEIGH LESS® WITH THE PEACE DIET

Weight Loss without Fighting Hunger

I just kept on eating and eating. And I never felt hungry and I lost 45 pounds.   Sharon W.

Would you like weight loss without having to battle your hunger drive? The Peace Diet is a simple way to accomplish that. Most diets put you at war with your hunger drive by forcing you to eat smaller portions than your body craves. The Peace Diet induces weight control by showing you how to choose foods that keep your body from having to fight your hunger drive and be at peace. In doing so, it makes weight control much easier and more sustainable in the long run. You will be at peace with your hunger drive. What is more important is that your body will be at peace metabolically so that the food that you consume will not cause a health battle within you. Here's an example of a comment from a participant in our Program

I never went away from the meal feeling hungry or deprived and that was one of the problems I've had with diets in the past because I've always had to eat a lot less food - but not with Dr. Shintani's diet. William G.

Automatic Weight Loss

Weight loss for people following the principles of the Peace Diet seems to come about automatically. When I myself first started eating this way, I lost 35 pounds without even thinking about it. The best part of it was that I didn't count calories or limit portion sizes, I didn't have to fight my hunger drive, and I lost weight even though I wasn't even trying to.

The reason for this automatic weight loss is simple: nature will not let you get fat if you eat whole, unprocessed food. If you choose foods according to the principles of the Peace Diet, you'll naturally move toward your ideal body weight because you are finally eating the food your body was designed to eat. This happens because whole foods - nature's foods - fill up your stomach before you can consume the excess calories that add up to extra pounds.

Eat As Much As You Want

One of the best parts of this approach is that you really can eat as much as you want! When I ask people, "What would you rather do? Eat less to lose weight, or eat more?" They always choose to eat more.

> *If somebody were to tell me that you could eat as much as you wanted and still lose weight, I wouldn't have believed it, but it's true. At every single meal I ate more than I normally would eat and I was never really hungry... and I still lost weight. And the cravings for the food that I had - for the foods you really shouldn't eat - seemed to disappear.* Gail M

> *I never ever felt deprived, and I've lost 37 pounds so far.*
> Karen T.

> *"I've lost 56 pounds and I've kept it off for 7 years."* Mary M.

An emphasis on whole, unprocessed food is a major reason the Peace Diet works. In fact, if you look at the number of pounds of food it takes to provide a day's worth of calories (which we will do later in this chapter), you'll realize why weight loss is automatic when you follow this way of eating.

The Lesson of the Apple and the Muffin

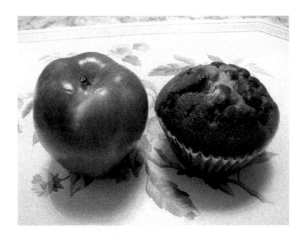

Above is a picture of two foods of approximately the same size and weight: an apple and a large muffin. Whenever I give a talk about the Peace Diet, the first question I ask of the audience is, "If you are hungry, could you eat two apples?"

Most people will answer yes to this question. Then I ask, "If you are hungry, could you eat two muffins?"

Again, the answer is usually yes. Most people can consume both these foods in similar quantities. Then I ask the audience if they can guess the number of calories in each food. I tell the audience that the apple is approximately 90 calories, and then ask, "Can you guess how many calories are in the muffin?" (Keep in mind that while the apple is whole and natural, the muffin is made of processed flour, processed sugar, processed oils-- and if it isn't homemade, probably several other chemicals.)

When I ask this question, most people answer somewhere between 250 to 350 calories. A few people boldly guess 400 calories. The reality is that the muffin provides a whopping 550 calories! This is usually surprising-- if not shocking-- to most people.

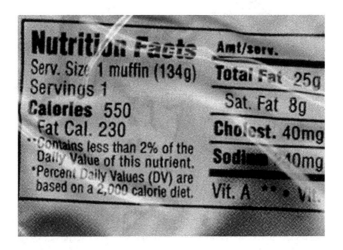

Putting this into context, think how many apples it takes to equal the calories of one muffin. Using simple math, you can calculate that it takes six apples to provide 540 calories (6 x 90 multiplies to 540), which means it takes 12 apples to equal the number of calories from two muffins. Most people can eat two muffins if they are hungry. I don't know any normal person who could eat 12 apples. They would get full long before they reached the 12th apple, which means they would feel fuller on far fewer calories.

As I said earlier, the profound lesson here is this: nature will not let you get fat! If you eat foods that are whole, natural, and plant-based, it is virtually impossible to consume enough calories to gain excess weight - even if you are eating a lot of food.

Natural Weight Control

In the late 1980s, when I pioneered the concept of how to eat more to lose weight, I trademarked the phrase "Eat More, Weigh Less®"[7] based on the idea that whole, unprocessed food provides more bulk with fewer calories, unlike many types of food we eat today, and is a sustainable way of maintaining health. The effectiveness of this approach, with its claim that people can eat more food but still wind up consuming fewer calories, has been published in peer-reviewed journals, where its short- and long-term effectiveness has been confirmed.[8] In addition, I have published seven years' worth of follow-up data showing that the long-term effectiveness of this approach is indeed sustainable.[9]

The idea for the Peace Diet approach to natural weight control began when I worked at a community health center, where most of my patients were Native Hawaiians. This is a population suffering from among the highest rates of obesity and obesity-related diseases in the world. I noticed that before the introduction of modernized ways of eating, the Native Hawaiians were slim and athletic. By sharp contrast, modern Hawaiians, like other Polynesian and some Native American populations, have very high rates of obesity and diabetes.

I figured that the obesity problem couldn't be simply genetic because ancient Hawaiian drawings and photographs showed these ancient peoples to be slim back when their genes were still purely Hawaiian, undiluted by the genes of newcomers. If obesity were genetic, then shouldn't those ancient Hawaiians have been more obese when their genes were still purely Native Hawaiian? I began to believe that, instead of a genetic cause, there must have been something about the diet of ancient Hawaiians that kept them slim.

The ancient Hawaiian diet consisted mainly of taro, poi (a pudding-like food made from taro), sweet potato, and yams – all starchy vegetables – but there were other types of vegetables as well, in addition to fruits, seaweed, and some seafood. Sugar, flour, and added oils weren't present at all.

Finding Foods That Cause Weight Loss

I'm thinking of measurements in grams, however, so I converted this calorie count into pounds, to show how many pounds of this particular food it would take to provide one day's worth of calories. The result was 5 pounds of poi. (This number is based on the estimation that 2500 calories a day is what an average-sized, inactive man, or an average-sized, active woman would need, in order to maintain his or her weight.)

These results aren't limited to poi, however. As another example, Native Hawaiians have traditionally also eaten sweet potatoes. By the same type of calculation, it would take about seven pounds of sweet potato to provide a day's worth of calories. Seven pounds!

By now, you may be thinking to yourself that most people can't eat five pounds of anything in a day, so they surely couldn't ever gain weight eating something like poi. Even if they ate until they were completely, utterly full, they wouldn't have taken in nearly enough calories to have added any extra pounds onto their bodies.

The point is, it was next to impossible for Native Hawaiians to become obese on their traditional mainstays, whether sweet potatoes or poi or any other foods, because of this fullness factor. Fortunately, this scenario isn't limited to ancient peoples, or traditional Hawaiian cuisine; it can be applied to any food culture, anywhere in the world.

High SMI (Food Mass Index) Foods Results in Low BMI (Body Mass Index)

To help other people learn to look at the relationship between food and fullness, I developed a table that I call the "Shintani Mass Index" (SMI) of food, a unique tool to help you determine which foods will help you feel full and still lose weight, and this tool was the key to the "Eat More Weigh Less®" Diet that I published years ago. It is like the mirror image to the "BMI" or Body Mass Index used to evaluate whether a person has a healthy weight for his or her height. The "SMI" is like a "Food Mass Index" that helps you evaluate whether a food has a healthy weight for the number of calories it contains. I call it a "mirror image" because the higher the SMI number in a food (i.e. the more a food weighs as compared to its caloric content), the lower your BMI (your weight to height ratio) will tend to be. In other words, a higher SMI number means a trimmer you.

As mentioned before, the SMI number represents the number of pounds of a selected food you would need to eat each day to consume your whole day's worth of calories, estimated at 2,500 cal.[10] A food with an SMI of 1.0 means you could only eat one pound of that food (if that were the only food you were going to eat all day), to reach 2,500 calories. A food with an SMI of 7.0 means you'd have to eat 7 lbs. of that food to reach the 2,500 calories, and that food would be a much more filling, better-for-you food choice.

Obviously, foods with lower SMIs have more calories per pound of food. They also tend to be less nutrient-dense. Conversely, foods with higher SMIs have fewer calories per pound, and more nutrients per calorie. They also have more vitamins, more antioxidants, more minerals, and greater anticancer nutrient values for every calorie you consume.

The Peace Diet Naturally Includes Foods That Cause Weight Loss

Through the lens of the SMI table, you start to see that the Peace Diet will help you choose foods that will induce natural weight loss. On the chart below are some examples of common foods. Notice that whole, unprocessed foods are all high on the SMI scale, while the typical American Diet foods all have low SMI numbers.

---

[10] 2,500 calories is a general guideline for the number of calories an average sedentary man or an average active woman requires each day to maintain their weight. This number is different for different people, depending on age, metabolism, activity level, and other factors. It is used here as a general dietary guideline, and enables the SMI to be standardized. It doesn't matter if your actual requirements are more or less than these numbers. This is simply a way to provide a rough idea which foods are likely to fill you up and help you to control your weight while satisfying hunger.

Comparison of Peace Diet Foods with American Diet Foods

Peace Diet	Grains:	SMI	Pounds Required for 2500 calories
	Brown Rice:	4.9	4.9
	Oatmeal	7.7	7.7
	Sweet Potato	5.4	5.4
	Baked Potato	5.9	5.9
American Diet			
	White Bread	2.1	2.1
	French Fries	1.7	1.7
	Potato Chips	1.0	1.0

Peace Diet	Vegetables	SMI	Pounds Required for 2500 calories
	Broccoli	17.1	17.1
	Tomato	27.3	27.3
	Kale	10.3	10.3
	Carrot	13.0	13.0
American Diet			
	Cole Slaw	3.6	3.6
	Mayonnaise	0.8	0.8
	Ranch Dressing	1.3	1.3

Peace Diet	Beans	SMI	Pounds Required for 2500 calories
	Black Beans	4.2	4.2
	Lima Beans	7.0	7.0
	Tofu	7.6	7.6
	Garbanzo Beans	4.0	4.0
American Diet			
	Ground Beef	1.9	1.9
	Fried Chicken	2.2	2.2
	Cheese	1.4	1.4
	Skinless Chicken Breast	3.8	3.8

Peace Diet	Fruit	SMI	Pounds Required for 2500 calories
	Apple	9.4	9.4
	Orange	15.6	15.6
	Strawberry	14.8	14.8
	Grapes	11.9	11.9
American Diet			
	Apple Pie	2.3	2.3
	Ice Cream	2.6	2.6
	Chocolate Cake	1.4	1.4
	Donut, glazed	1.3	1.3

Quantities of Food Required to Provide 2500 Calories

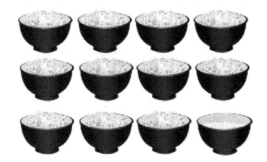

11.5 Bowls of Rice (4.9 lbs)

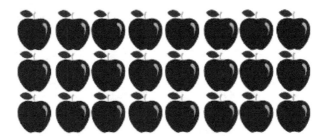

24 medium Apples (9.6 lbs)

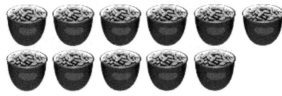

11 Cups of Kidney Beans (4.2 lbs)

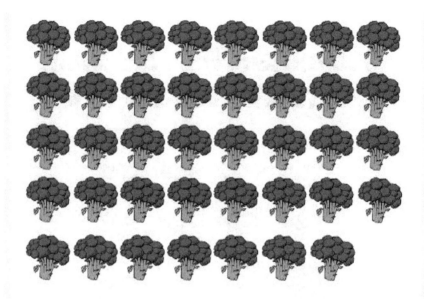

39 heads of broccoli, (17.1 pounds; 2,500 Calories)

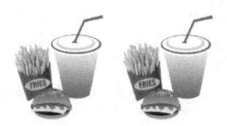

**2 Burgers, 2 medium french Fries and
2 medium drinks
(1.9 pounds of food
and two 20 oz drinks, 2,500 Calories)**

As you look at these foods and familiarize yourself with their SMI numbers, you will see that the foods from the Peace Diet all have moderate to high numbers. Most people, when allowed to eat without restriction, will eat no more than 2.6 to 4.1 pounds per day. [11] [12] This means that there is really no way to gain excess weight when following the Peace Diet, because virtually all of its foods will fill you up long before you get enough calories to even maintain your weight. You wind up losing weight automatically.

Let's look at oatmeal as an example. Oatmeal has an SMI value of 7.7. That means if you were going to eat only oatmeal for a day (though I'm not suggesting you do that), you would need to eat 7.7 pounds of it to reach your day's total of 2,500 calories. (Remember that 2,500 calories is an estimate based on an average inactive man or an active woman. Your daily requirement might be slightly different.) I don't know about you, but I couldn't imagine eating that much oatmeal, no matter how much I love it! Even if you did plan to eat nothing but oatmeal for a day, you probably couldn't even eat half that much. You would feel overly, uncomfortably full.

By contrast, if you eat foods from the standard American diet, it is easy to eat bread and hamburger and cheese and still feel hungry at the end of the day. This is because these foods are so concentrated in calories that it doesn't take much of them to provide a whole lot of calories. As a result, their SMI numbers are small. In other words, it would take less than 2 or 3 pounds of these types of food to provide your entire day's worth of calories, which could easily leave room in your stomach and cause you to eat more than your day's allotment of calories. The result would be weight gain, and often you'd still be feeling hungry all the time.

Lose Weight While Eating More Food

Food mass helps you feel full and satisfied. So choosing foods based on the SMI chart by looking for foods that have a higher SMI value helps you to control your weight while eating as much as you want. Our studies show that calorie intake automatically decreases with foods that have more mass per calorie. The higher the number, the more you can eat per calorie. When the numbers are high enough, there is no way to gain weight and weight loss can become automatic for those who are overweight. Our studies show that calorie intake goes down even while eating more food. This is why it is called the "Eat More, Weigh Less®" diet concept.

Eat More to Weigh Less

Food Intake and Calorie Intake on High SMI Diet vs. Modern American Diet

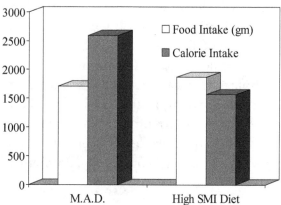

Shintani TT.
Am J Clin Nutr 1991; 53: 1647S-51S.

Peace Diet and Weight Control

The Peace Diet emphasizes five additional aspects of food that will help you lose weight. The SMI chart also helps you identify the foods that have these qualities.

1. Whole Plant-Based Food

Overall, the Peace Diet encourages you to eat whole plant-based foods which not coincidentally tend to be high on the SMI scale. These are the foods that are naturally high in fiber, low in fat, high in water content, and high in vitamin, mineral, and micronutrient content. These characteristics, which I describe individually below, automatically contribute to health and ideal weight.

Conversely, foods that are low on the SMI scale tend to be either processed or based on commercially raised animal products. For example, you will notice that foods that are not whole and are highly refined foods such as sugar, white flour, and oils, (people forget that oil is a highly processed food) are very low on the SMI. Not only do they not fill up your stomach and leave you hungry, they are devoid of the nutrients that can help optimize health.

Flour products, which are not whole in that they are milled, tend to be lower on the SMI than un-milled grain such as brown rice. Be careful, however, because flour products such as pastries are laden with fat and sugar and are low on the SMI and will contribute to your weight gain very quickly.

Avoiding animal products is also helpful in contributing to weight control. Most animal products are low on the SMI scale because they tend to be quite high in fat. In fact, keeping the fat low is another way the Peace Diet helps with natural weight control.

2. Minimum Fat

A major factor in the Peace Diet is its low fat content. Fundamentally, fat is an important factor that causes people to be fat and percent fat in the food you eat roughly determines the percent of fat on your body.

Studies on mice are consistent with this effect. Researchers at the University of Massachusetts fed groups of genetically similar mice feed of various percentages of fat in them and let them eat as much as they wanted. After a few months, they measured the body fat of the mice. They found that the higher the fat content of the food, the higher the body fat of the mice and that the rate of obesity increased from 0% with the low fat diet to 35% with the high fat diet.

Dietary Fat and Body Fat

More dietary fat is associated with more body fat

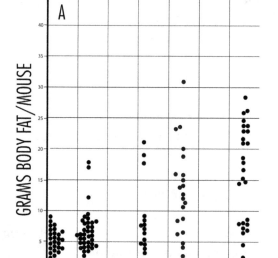

Percent Fat in Non-Calorie-Restricted Diet

Adapted from: Salmon D, Flatt J; Int J Obes (1985); 9(6)443.

Notice that this research supports the idea that the Peace Diet will support natural control of body fat even while eating as much as you want. You will find that almost all the foods that are high in SMI are also very low in fat and vice-versa.

Animal products tend also to be high in fat and low on the SMI scale. For example, beef is typically 65% to 70% fat. Pork is typically about the same. Processed meats are higher with luncheon meat, bologna and sausages at about 83% fat and bacon at about 90% fat. Chicken is around 46% to 60% fat. Dairy is also typically high in fat. Whole milk is about 55% fat, and 2% milk is actually 35% fat. Cheese is around 76% fat.

Whole, unprocessed food tends to be low in fat. For example, potatoes are very low in fat at less than 2%. Their SMI value is around 5.9, so it takes 5.9 pounds of potatoes to provide 2500 calories. Potato chips by contrast are nearly 60% fat and it takes just 1 pound of potato chips to provide 2500 calories. These are examples of how the Peace Diet naturally provides a low fat way of eating that helps keep weight under control. Later, you will see that reducing fat intake also helps to control cholesterol and inflammation.

3. Minimum Processed Carbohydrate

Foods high in processed carbohydrates tend to be low on the SMI scale, so choosing foods that are high on the SMI scale conversely are low in processed carbohydrates. This is important because, as described in the section on health below, processed carbohydrates contribute to elevated insulin levels. Insulin is a hormone that helps to control blood sugar, but it also contributes to weight gain, high blood sugar, high blood pressure, and high cholesterol.

Thus, by following the Peace Diet you will be avoiding foods that will contribute to "metabolic syndrome" as described in the next chapter. The Peace Diet will also help you to choose good carbohydrate foods that help to reduce the risk of heart disease, cancer and stroke. Remember that the countries that consume the most carbohydrates have the lowest levels of these diseases. The important factor for these populations is that they don't consume much fat or many processed carbohydrates.

4. Maximum Fiber

Fiber is one of the main substances that make high SMI foods high in SMI. Fiber tends to hold water and does so without calories. In other words, it provides satisfaction without adding weight. Fiber also helps to prevent heart disease, stomach cancer, colon cancer and constipation.

5. Maximum Micronutrients

Whole foods also contain a wide variety of micronutrients such as vitamins and minerals. Though we may never completely understand how our bodies utilize all the micronutrients found in whole foods, we do know beyond a doubt that our bodies were designed to use the micronutrients found in natural foods. Recent scientific data increasingly supports the wisdom of eating whole foods because many of the substances found in whole foods may reduce the risk of cancer and heart disease, and help your immune system, which is vital to health.

For example, substances such as beta carotene, retinoids, vitamin C, vitamin E, flavonoids, triterpenoids, polyphenols, cathechins and selenium, to name a few, have antioxidant and anti-inflammatory properties that may help prevent cancer and cardiovascular disease. These and so many of the other substances found only in whole foods are essential ingredients in any eating program if we are ever to function at maximum capacity, ward off disease, and maintain our ideal weight.

The fundamental Eat More, Weigh Less® principle works for just about anyone. If you eat high SMI foods, primarily whole foods, you'll eat bulkier, more filling foods. You'll feel satisfied, you'll begin to lose weight with no effort other than choosing the right foods, and eventually you'll achieve your ideal weight -- without feeling deprived! So the thing to do is focus on changing your foods, rather than driving yourself mad by trying to cut down on the foods you eat. Or, said another way, if you'll just start eating the right foods, you don't have to worry about the amounts you eat. You can reach your ideal body weight naturally because your hunger drive will be satisfied and at peace.

Making Peace with Your Cravings

Cravings are an issue that comes up with any dietary change. This is the result of a combination of pure habit and some primordial physiology. Participants in my 10-Day Program say that their cravings are much easier to control after following the diet for several days. Let me explain why I think this happens, so you can have a better handle on your cravings.

Before I started a vegetarian diet when I was 26 years old, I used to like to take my dates to a steak house. I happened to know one of the singers who entertained there, and I wanted to impress my date that I had "connections." I used to start off with a small salad with a lot of thousand-island dressing on it. Then I would order a 12 oz prime rib, well done, with baked potato and dinner rolls. I would slather the potato in butter and sprinkle it with salt, and I would eat several rolls, also well-buttered. This could easily add up to close to 2500 calories and be nearly as many calories as I needed for the whole day. The interesting thing is that even after eating all that, I still craved ice cream. Modern science can't really explain why a person who has had that many calories would still crave more food.

There's a surprisingly simple and useful explanation for this phenomenon from the Macrobiotic approach to dietary recommendations. Macrobiotics is a word used by Hippocrates meaning "long (macro) life (bios)." The founder of Macrobiotics, Georges Ohsawa, adopted this word to describe his philosophy of life and healing which is based on Chinese medicine principles as practiced in Japan with a major emphasis on food as a pathway to health and happiness. Ohsawa's greatest student and proponent was Micho Kushi, who was my teacher.

Part of understanding of Macrobiotics is appreciating the ever-changing balance between yin and yang, the two major energies in the physical manifestation of the world. Yin is the female, soft and expansive energy of things. Yang is the male, firm and contractive energy of things. Yin attracts yang and yang attracts yin.

Food has these characteristics as well. Salt, meat, and baked goods are foods that are very yang in nature. Fruit, sweets, dairy and alcohol are yin in nature. So when one eats a lot of food that is yang in nature, craving yin is a natural result despite getting enough calories. Thus, from this perspective, eating lots of meat and salt causes craving of sweets and alcohol. So it is obvious that eating a steak will induce the desire for dessert and a drink.

Science hasn't really caught up with these concepts because cravings are a difficult thing to measure. However, in my Program, people consistently say that their cravings are much easier to handle after changing their diet. Some of this occurs because the diet is full of nutrients that support good health, and so there is no starving for missing nutrients. Some of it may be explained by some ancient concepts of the energy of food. It makes sense that in the Peace Diet, the extremes of "yin" and "yang" foods are eliminated, and a balance in the food is more easily achieved. Meat, animal products, salt, and baked goods are limited as well as sugar, dairy and alcohol. As a result, an easy balance is formed and cravings are diminished.

Of course, some cravings come up at one point or another in everyone. This is where the SMI becomes useful. For example, if you crave something sweet, instead of grabbing a cookie or a piece of candy, choose a piece of fruit or a slice of sweet potato. Also incorporate some sweet vegetables such as squash or carrots into your cooking. If you crave something salty, instead of potato chips, try some garbanzo beans rinsed of the salty water that they are packed in. They are like boiled peanuts but with much less fat. I like "Eden" brand for the beans that they pack in seaweed (kelp) water which would provide for some trace minerals to be in it. Also some brown rice flavored with seaweed sprinkles or Bragg's Liquid Aminos® would be a good choice. In any case, choosing foods that are higher on the SMI scale will help you to make choices that will help you deal with cravings and still control your weight.

Peace Diet Principles of Weight Control
So, by using the SMI table and following the guidelines of the Peace Diet, you can see that it will help you lose weight naturally, without the need to count every calorie. The principles of the Peace Diet will help you choose foods that fill you up before you can get enough calories to gain weight. Also remember that I mentioned at the beginning of this book, food alone isn't what leads you to healthy weight and good health overall. Eating foods that follow the principles of the Peace Diet will truly help to elevate your spirit, will also be truly healthy for your mind and body, and will be your best path to a healthy weight.

The Peace Diet recommends the following:

1. Eat According to the Peace Plate (Whole, unprocessed plant-based)
2. Eat foods that are higher on the SMI scale
3. Eat according to the season (when possible) and to your locality
4. Chew your food well: 25 times per mouthful
5. Slow down or stop eating when 80% full, so that satiety can catch up
6. Don't eat within three hours of going to bed
7. Eat for balance in order to curb cravings
8. Remember the eight enhancements to the Peace Diet

The Peace Diet is Flexible

As a final note, the Peace Diet is not meant to be followed in a rigid manner except in periods of a focused spiritual quest. I think the diet should be tailored to individual needs and circumstances. It is not a one diet fits all. It should be adjusted to climate, season, and one's constitution. If a person is allergic or sensitive to certain foods, then, of course such foods should be avoided. It is perfectly natural on occasion to allow for party food at celebrations. The important thing is to go right back to the principles of the Peace Diet to maintain your good health.

I don't expect everyone to be vegetarian even though I think it is ideal and better for the health of people and the world. The reality is that most cultures did consume small amounts of meat. If flesh is consumed, I recommend that appropriate prayers be said to acknowledge the taking of a life for food. This may help to reduce the karmic debt related to the death and suffering of the animal.

I also recommend against consuming farm-raised animals because they are in general not treated well and they are fattened-up naturally and unnaturally. This typically changes the fat quality and quantity. For example, wild game is roughly 20% in fat Calorie percentage. Typical cuts of commercially produced meat is around 60% to 70% in fat calorie percentage. In addition, the fat of wild animals has a higher proportion of omega 3 fats in it. This is because it is eating natural plant based food instead of commercial feed. Even meat-eaters can benefit by following the Peace Diet because the longest lived people rarely ate meat and did not do so daily. Thus, in order to model after such populations, even a meat-eater or omnivore would have to learn how to eat whole plant-based foods for the days they are not eating meat.

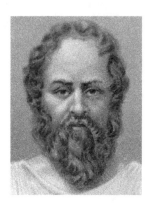

"The highest realms of thought are impossible to reach without first attaining an understanding of compassion."
-SOCRATES (469-399 B.C.)

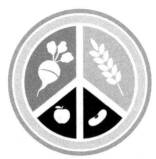

IV- REVERSE AGING AND DISEASE WITH THE PEACE DIET

"Any animal that gets old enough, will get the pathology of Alzheimers - except for herbivores." [13] Rudoph Tanzi, PhD, Harvard Neuroscientist and Alzheimer's Expert

In our 10-day programs, individuals have seen their biological age reduced by as much as 11 years in just 10 days. This is based on biological markers including blood pressure, serum cholesterol, blood sugar, weight, and activity.[14] We all have a chronological age and a biological age. Our biological age is based on a number of factors. Probably the most important factor is the health and condition of our bodies. We can't change time, but we can change our bodies and our health.

Part of the reason the Peace Diet may help to reverse the aging process is because it helps to reduce the intensity of the many battles your body is fighting. Bringing peace to your body's metabolic processes may reduce your disease burden and reduce your risk of disability and death. This is one of the keys to good health as we age because one of the main factors that cause aging is inflammation caused by the lack of peace in your bodily functions. The Peace Diet may contribute to vibrant longevity in several ways.

Calorie Control

There has long been evidence that calorie restriction can consistently increase life-span.[15]   This effect has been seen across species all the way from worms to mammals.   In the previous chapter, you can see how this diet can naturally reduce calorie intake even while eating enough food to feel full and satisfied. Because of this effect, the Peace Diet naturally contributes to longevity in this basic way.

Less Methionine

In addition, in recent studies, it has been suggested that the reduction in the intake of an essential amino acid, methionine, may have the same effect on longevity as calorie restriction without having to restrict calories.[16] This apparent effect on life-span is thought to be a result of the pro-oxidant effect of methionine. Animal products are quite high in methionine; plant-based proteins are very adequate but much lower in methionine content. For this reason, some researchers believe that following a plant-based diet may be one way to contribute to healthy anti-aging effects.[17]

The avoidance of animal products in the Peace Diet may be one of the factors that also contributes to longevity. In a review of six large population studies, it appears that less meat means more years of life expectancy This may be because less meat means less methionine intake.

Less Obesity

Obesity is a risk factor for numerous diseases and is one of the factors commonly used to determine health age. Of course, the higher the weight to height ratio (calculated as "Body Mass Index" or BMI) the higher the mortality from many diseases. Some of the many diseases associated with obesity are, heart disease, cancer, high blood pressure stroke, diabetes, arthritis, sleep apnea, autoimmune disease, and many more chronic health conditions. The Peace Diet describes how to control obesity in the previous chapter even while eating more food.

Less Heart Disease

It makes sense that a reduction in obesity and meat consumption and an increase in whole plant-based food as recommended in the Peace Diet should help to increase your life-span. This is because meat consumption is associated with increases in the risk of heart disease, and stroke, two of the three leading causes of death.

People following the recommendations of the Peace Diet consistently notice a reduction in cholesterol, triglycerides, LDL, and non-HDL cholesterol.   There is also a consistent improvement in blood pressure even in two or three days. In fact, the improvement is so rapid that some participants have to reduce their blood pressure medication in as little as two days.
The reasons for the reduction of risk of these diseases are detailed in the chapter on heart disease.

Less Inflammation

Inflammation is the key to most of the chronic diseases suffered in later years. In fact some experts report that virtually all chronic diseases of aging have an inflammatory component. The conditions associated with inflammation are similar to the ones associated with obesity. This should be no surprise since obesity itself causes inflammation in the body. These conditions include heart disease, cancer, diabetes, neurological diseases, Alzheimers's disease, arthritis, chronic pain, autoimmune disease, allergy, and much more. In our Peace Diet program, markers for inflammation generally go down and pain scores improve consistently.

We have even seen very difficult cases improved, sometimes dramatically such as rheumatoid arthritis, uncreative colitis, psoriasis and other autoimmune diseases that are supposedly incurable. See Chapter VI on "How to bring peace to the inflammation in your body.

Control of Blood Sugar

The control of blood sugar and diabetes is now at the forefront of modern medicine. This is because of the alarming news that nearly half of all Americans have abnormal blood sugar. This is of crucial importance because high blood sugar leads to the damage of small blood vessels throughout the body and poor circulation in many vital organs. In the U.S., diabetes is the leading cause of blindness, kidney dialysis, and below the knee amputations. Diabetes also contributes to heart disease, impotence (erectile dysfunction), neuropathy, incontinence, stroke, dementia, and Alzheimer's disease. In fact, some people call Alzheimer's disease "diabetes of the brain". See chapter VII for more information on controlling diabetes and blood sugar even while eating more carbs.

Controlling Cancer

Cancer is poised to become the leading cause of death in America. According the National Cancer Institute, in their "Surveillance, Epidemiology, and End Results" database, researchers predict that one in two men will get cancer and one in three women will get cancer at some time in their lives. Cancer is actually already the number one cause of death in several states. The scary thing is that in 1971, it is estimated that cancer struck only one out of 21 people. Surely, learning how to prevent and remove factors that cause cancer to grow is an important lesson to learn. Chapter VIII on cancer covers this topic.

Anti-oxidation

Some experts think of aging as the gradual oxidation of our bodies -- similar to how oxidation causes metal to rust. One reason that the Peace Diet may help to extend your life is because the large amounts of vegetables and fruit recommended are full of anti-oxidant substances. Much of this is covered in Chapter XIII on the description of the "Peace Plate".

Reducing Your Need for Medication

The 4th leading cause of death in the U.S. may be prescription medication according to a stunning report in the Journal of the American Medical Association.[18] I'm not saying pharmaceuticals are not useful. What I am saying is that they never make you truly healthy and always risk side-effects. I always remind people that if they are on prescription medication, by definition, they are still sick. Part of the reason is that artificial chemicals never truly bring peace to your body. It may fix one battle here or there, but it always causes a battle in some other way. This is because in consuming an unnatural chemical, your body has to deal with a substance that is foreign to it, and it is a battle for your body. And in doing so, it upsets the harmony of your body's functions.

This is why it is important to eat in a way that brings peace to your body. When it is at peace, it functions in a healthy way and then you minimize your need for medication. Then you are able to put fewer artificial chemicals (drugs) into your body and in doing so, you further bring peace to your body. This is one of the important outcomes of following the Peace Diet. In our Program, using the Peace Diet, we have seen an estimated reduction in the cost of medication of approximately 24% in just 10 days.

Heartburn

Battles in the body are early indicators that you are not totally healthy and that something needs to change. Heartburn is a good example of a battle that is going on in your body, telling you that something is not right with your body. One of the most commonly prescribed types of medications in the U.S. is heartburn medicine. In 2013, Nexium®, was number 2 in sales. You've probably also seen Tagamet®, Prilosec®, and other prescription and over-the-counter drugs for treating heartburn in the store or on television commercials, where the spokespeople talk about how you take just one pill and then eat all the foods you want without experiencing any more heartburn.

The problem with medications such as these is that it's like there is a fire going on in your stomach, and your answer is to turn off the alarm instead of putting out the fire. When you experience heartburn, your body is telling you something is not right, that you are eating the wrong food, or overeating, or eating at the wrong time, such as too close to bedtime. From jaw to tooth to digestive system, humans are built more similar to herbivores than to carnivores or even omnivores (see the later chapter "Anatomy of Peace" for more about this.) Based on previous USDA recommendations, we were encouraged to eat meat three times a day and to eat lots of protein. Problem was, when we ate more meat and protein, our stomachs put out lots of acid because acid is needed to digest animal products.

Because our digestive tracts are built more like those of herbivores, we are not accustomed to such large amounts of acid unless we have lots of plant-type material in our stomach -- in other words, lots of fiber. Fiber is the non-digestible part of plants that holds water in your stomach, keeps stool matter bulky, and dilutes the acid. If you don't have adequate fiber in your stomach, and all you do is eat meat, processed flour, and dairy – for example a cheeseburger on a bun – then you have lots of acid production but virtually no fiber to hold onto water to dilute the acid. Thus, your stomach becomes inflamed, and you feel heartburn.

A simple solution to most of the cases of heartburn is the Peace Diet. (There are other health problems with symptoms that can resemble heartburn. If you have persistent symptoms that feel like heartburn, you should see your doctor to make sure it isn't something more serious.) When you consume lots of whole grains, vegetables, fruits, and beans, the fiber that is inherent in those types of foods will protect your stomach from its own acid. In contrast, when you eat something like pizza with pepperoni, you're getting two parts of this problem at once: a large amount of protein from the meat and cheese, plus too little fiber because most of it has been processed out from the white-flour crust. You have then eaten acid-producing foods, but eaten nothing to neutralize that acid, which creates an acid stomach and heartburn.

The other solution to heartburn relates to taste. Most people know that the taste of acidity is sour – you're probably familiar with vinegar or citric acids from sour fruits like lemons. However, most people are less familiar with the taste of alkaline, which is bitter. Yet alkalinity neutralizes acid. When you eat bitter greens such as dandelion greens, you are preventing heartburn. Eating vegetables, and chewing them up well enough to get the juice into your stomach, helps combat heartburn in two ways: by bringing alkalizing properties into the gut, and by contributing fiber. So, by eating plenty of vegetable matter and by cutting down consumption of meat, dairy and white flour products - just as the Peace Diet recommends, you may find that your heartburn disappears.

General Health and Well Being

Numerous conditions may improve with the Peace Diet, including overall energy, heart disease, diabetes, hypertension, insomnia, skin conditions, inflammation, chronic pain, digestive, and many others I have heard patients report. This wide range of health conditions that improves is a result of eating and behaving in a way to bring peace to the body's metabolic processes.

In general, the health of most people will be enhanced if they follow the Peace Diet. Individuals do vary, of course, and people with special health conditions should seek the guidance of their primary care physician before changing their diet dramatically. This is especially true for those who are on medication; for some people, health may improve so quickly that their medication dosage becomes too strong, even dangerous. This is an indication of how effective the Peace Diet can be! In the next several chapters, we will describe several specific conditions and ways in which the Peace Diet has been shown to be helpful.

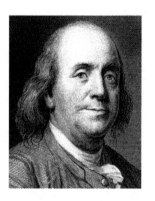

*"My refusing to eat meat occasioned
inconveniency, and I have been frequently
chided for my singularity. But my light
repast allows for greater progress, for
greater clearness of head and quicker
comprehension."
-BENJAMIN FRANKLIN (1706-1790)*

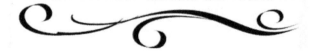

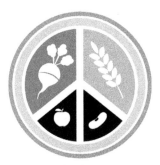

V-WINNING THE CHOLESTEROL AND HEART DISEASE BATTLE

"My cholesterol used to be 223. Now, about two years later, it's 131." Margaret F.

If you win the battle with cholesterol, you are likely to improve your life expectancy a great deal because cholesterol is connected to the leading cause of death in the world. The number one killer in the world is cardiovascular disease, especially heart attack and stroke. There are many risk-factors that may contribute to cardiovascular disease such as smoking, obesity, diabetes, hypertension, family history, insulin levels, lack of exercise, and others. Two keys to controlling these diseases lie in controlling cholesterol, especially LDL or the "bad cholesterol," and in controlling inflammation. The Peace Diet helps to control both.

If you are on cholesterol medication in the category known as "statins" you may want to eliminate or reduce your need for these medications. This is important because the side-effects of "statins" may include memory loss, muscle damage, and liver damage. It would be better to control your cholesterol with fewer of these medications. Here is an example of a comment from one of the participants in our Program.

When I started the program, my cholesterol level was around 235, and it went down 100 points in three weeks. I'm telling you, I was astounded. I've been trying to get that cholesterol down for years and years and it's never been that low. And here it is. All I had to do was change my diet . . . and basically follow what Dr. Shintani said to do. And it works, and it works fast. And that was incredible.
Robert G.

Cholesterol and Heart Disease

Most people are aware that high cholesterol levels in the blood are a risk factor for heart disease. The fact that animal fat and cholesterol promote atherosclerosis which leads to cardiovascular disease has been demonstrated in animal and human studies. It was demonstrated in primates that a diet that is higher in butter, lard and cholesterol promoted atherosclerosis, and a diet that was low in these substances did not.[19] In human studies, researchers demonstrated that a low-fat plant-based diet could induce a reversal of atherosclerosis.[20]

There has been a controversy about whether cholesterol actually causes heart disease because of some recent correlational studies that suggest that there is no relationship between cholesterol levels and heart disease while other studies indicate the opposite. However, correlational studies do not necessarily mean causation or lack thereof. Clinical studies such as the above-cited studies are really the gold standard and make any population studies that might suggest otherwise irrelevant in actual practice. In other words, based on numerous clinical studies, it has been shown that eating animal fat such as that which is found in lard, butter, and egg yolks promotes atherosclerosis or hardening and narrowing of arteries. They have also shown that removing these animal fats from the diet can induce a reduction in cholesterol and a reversal of atherosclerosis in animal and human studies.

Many people are aware that cholesterol is found only in animal-based foods. There is no cholesterol in plant-based foods; therefore, the basic Peace Diet has no cholesterol in it. However, the issue is not as simple as avoiding cholesterol. Overall fat intake is even more important to blood cholesterol than the intake of cholesterol by itself, so in order to prevent heart disease, it is important to control both fat intake and cholesterol intake.

The Peace Diet takes care of fat and cholesterol intake by providing a diet that naturally limits fat intake because of its plant-based food sources. One of my professors at Harvard University, Dr. William Castelli, is the former director of the Framingham Study, a long-term, ongoing cardiovascular study on residents of the town of Framingham, Massachusetts begun in 1948. Dr. Castelli is known as one of the great pioneers in the field of diet and heart disease, and his research has much to do with our current understanding of cholesterol, HDL, LDL, and heart disease. In a radio interview in 2011 on "Staying Healthy Today" radio, Dr. Castelli indicated that heart disease disappears when cholesterol levels get very low:

> *Now, if I would have put everyone on a vegetarian diet and drive their numbers down by diet, we would get rid of all the atherosclerosis in America.*

Dr. T. Colin Campbell, professor emeritus of Cornell University, conducted another long-term study called "The China Study," which has been hailed as the "Grand Prix" of all epidemiological studies on diet and health. [22]   Dr. Campbell states that,

Based on the findings (of this study), there appears to be no threshold for the benefits of eating plants. The greater the plant intake, the better the health benefits. . .[22]

In other words, the greatest health benefits come from a diet that is all natural whole plant-based food and zero animal products in it whatsoever. The "Peace Diet" is completely in line with Dr. Campbell's and Dr. Castelli's conclusions. By eliminating animal products and following the Peace Diet Plate as a guideline, you can reap a wide range of health benefits.

Other professionals have had similar findings. Dr. John McDougall, internist, author and founder of the McDougall Program has been successfully controlling cholesterol and blood pressure in patients by placing them on a plant-based diet for years. [23]   Dr. Caldwell Esselstyn, a cardiac surgeon and co-star of the "Forks over Knives" documentary with T. Colin Campbell, also demonstrated that a low-fat, high-carbohydrate plant-based diet could prevent and even reverse heart disease.[24]   In addition, the landmark "Lifestyle Heart Trial" showed regression of coronary artery disease with a 10% fat, high-carbohydrate vegetarian diet, while the control group, placed on a 30% fat Heart Association style diet which was lower in carbohydrates, showed a worsening of the cholesterol plaques.[25]

High Blood Pressure

I've lost 52 pounds, and I don't have to take blood pressure medicine anymore and my blood pressure stays normal
Ruth P.

Reversing the cholesterol plaque formation in the arteries also contributes to the reversal of high blood pressure. High blood pressure is another risk factor for heart disease. High blood pressure is also a risk factor for stroke and kidney failure. It is related to heart disease, partly because one of the causes of high blood pressure is hardening of the arteries. The arteries are hardened by the beginnings of the formation of cholesterol plaque in the arteries that lead to heart disease. When the arteries become hard and the opening of the artery narrowed by cholesterol plaque, it is like putting your thumb on the end of a hose. The pressure goes up because more pressure is needed to get liquid through a smaller opening than it is to get it through a bigger opening.

Keeping your blood cholesterol low ultimately has the potential of reversing the cholesterol plaque formation and the narrowing of the arteries caused by the cholesterol. When a whole plant-based diet is followed, cholesterol can be reduced enough that the plaques start to soften up and regress. This can allow the diameter of the artery to open up. Here again, the Peace Diet will help reduce the stiffness of the arteries. This in turn may help to reduce high blood pressure, underlying causes of high blood pressure, and also help to keep it permanently low over time.

High blood pressure is consistently brought under better control when people follow the guidelines of the "Peace Diet." Many previous program participants have managed to lower their blood pressure so much that medication requirements are reduced in as little as two or three days. We have had participants start the program with blood pressures of 190/110, and wind up with blood pressures in the 120's/80's. Here are some comments from participants themselves:

> *My blood pressure - you know when we first started out, I think the reading was 160/90. This morning, [21 days later], I monitored my blood pressure and went down to 124/64, and this is without the medication. Fred K.*

"Five days after the [start of Dr. Shintani's Program] my blood pressure medicine was completely stopped." Kay B.

"I have high blood pressure . . . In 3 days I got off my high blood pressure medicine. . ." Kathy P.

Part of the reason blood pressures improve on my Peace Diet Program is because most of the major sources of excess dietary sodium are eliminated, without sacrificing taste. According to the CDC (Centers for Disease Control), only 6% of sodium in a typical American Diet is added at the table-- and only 5% during home cooking. So, where is the rest of that dietary sodium coming from? It comes from processed foods. According to the CDC, here are the top 10 sources of sodium in the standard American Diet. [27]

Top 10 Sources of Sodium

1. Bread and rolls, 7.4%
2. Cold cuts/cured meats, 5.1%
3. Pizza, 4.9%
4. Fresh and processed poultry, 4.5%
5. Soups, 4.3%
6. Sandwiches like cheeseburgers, 4%
7. Cheese, 3.8%
8. Pasta dishes like spaghetti with meat sauce, 3.3%
9. Meat dishes like meatloaf with tomato sauce, 3.2%
10. Snacks, including chips, pretzels, popcorn and puffs, 3.1%

Minerals

In addition to naturally reducing sodium intake, the Peace Diet is high in nutrients that help to control blood pressure, such as potassium and magnesium, both of which play a vital role in aintaining cardiovascular health. Vegetables and fruit are typically high in both potassium and magnesium. In some cases, blood pressure may improve simply because a mineral deficiency has been corrected by the conversion to a plant-based diet rich in these mineral regulators.

Nitric Oxide

Another nutrient that helps to maintain healthy blood pressure is nitric oxide, which relaxes blood vessels, keeping blood pressure down. [27] (This is the same substance used in emergency medicine to open up blood vessels when a patient is experiencing chest pain.) Plant-based foods are full of substances that raise nitric oxide levels; some good examples of foods rich in these substances are beets, kale, oranges, brown rice, walnuts, and black tea. Following the Peace Diet guidelines and eating a wide variety of these types of foods will help ensure that you have good levels of nitric oxide in your blood stream to help keep your blood pressure at healthy levels.

Insulin

Earlier, the role of insulin and its relationship to blood sugar was discussed, but did you know it also plays a role in regulating blood pressure? Insulin causes blood pressure to rise because it makes blood vessels constrict. Thus, lowering insulin levels by following an insulin-controlling diet such as the Peace Diet will reduce vaso-constriction and keep blood pressure lower. This then reduces one major factor of those complex health conditions that make up "Metabolic Syndrome." These include obesity, high blood sugar, high triglycerides, and high blood pressure.

Reversing the Hardening of the Arteries

In the programs I myself conduct, cholesterol, blood pressure, and blood sugar are carefully tracked for a period of 10 to 21 days, depending on the program. In every group, there is a significant lowering of these cardiovascular disease markers. Some of my patients see their cholesterol decrease over 70 points in just 10 days, and over 100 points in just 21 days.

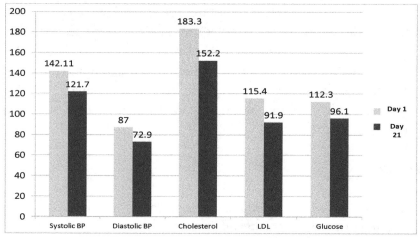

Dr. Shintani's "Peace Diet" Results

Other Factors Related to Heart Disease

There are other factors that contribute to the prevention of heart disease and all atherosclerotic cardiovascular disease besides cholesterol. Over the years, researchers have found that factors such as oxidation, inflammation, insulin, trans fats, and an amino acid known as homocysteine, all may play a role in heart disease. The Peace Diet helps your body to deal with all of these factors in different ways.

Oxidation contributes to heart disease when it occurs in LDL, the "bad" cholesterol. Oxidation of LDL may be induced, for example, by smoking, by exposure to free radicals, and by consuming over-heated oils. These oxidized LDL cholesterol particles trigger a response by the white blood cells to capture these particles and take them into the artery walls. This triggers inflammation and scarring of the artery walls.

Inflammation is what causes scar tissue to form on the inside of arteries that later becomes the cholesterol deposits that block arteries and cause heart disease and strokes. Heart disease rates tend to correlate to CRP or "C-Reactive Protein" which is a blood marker that indicates inflammation. A decrease in CRP is correlated to a decreased risk of heart disease.

The Peace Diets helps to control inflammation in several ways. The foods in the Peace Diet are full of anti-inflammatory nutrients that help to prevent heart disease and strokes. One of these nutrients called resveratrol is found in grapes. It is considered to be the reason behind the "French Paradox" in which people in France seem to have a relatively low rate of heart disease even though they consume a high fat diet. For more detail about the anti-inflammatory effects of the Peace Diet, go to the section below on inflammation in this chapter.

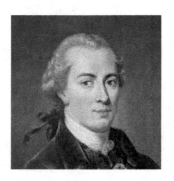

*"We can judge the heart of a man
by his treatment of animals."
-IMMANUEL KANT (1724-1804)*

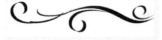

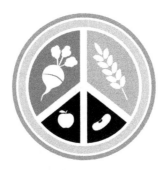

VI- BRINGING PEACE TO THE INFLAMMATION IN YOUR BODY

"I had a problem with my aches and pains and I don't know what happened to them. They're gone now." Joseph R.

Inflammation is the most classic and most common battle that is raging in your body. It is your body either fighting to protect itself from something or working to repair any damage that may have occurred. Some experts now say that all chronic disease is based on inflammation. This may be too broad a statement, but clearly the vast majority of chronic health conditions have an inflammatory component.

First, we must remember that inflammation is necessary for our health; inflammation helps our bodies ward off invasion by foreign and toxic materials such as poisons, foreign substances, bacteria, and viruses. It does so by calling up your body's defensive army of white blood cells to attack any invasion and defend your body. It is also an important factor in repairing damaged tissue by recruiting blood, oxygen, and white blood cells to disinfect and repair wounds. That said, it is true that inflammation is indeed tied to many diseases including heart and cardiovascular disease, as well as the more common and obvious conditions such as osteoarthritis, rheumatoid arthritis, back pain, neck pain, asthma, fibromyalgia, chronic fatigue, chronic pain, ulcerative colitis, allergy, auto-immune diseases, myasthenia gravis, and lupus.

Interestingly, all these diseases are more common in developed countries, where more fat and meat are consumed. Conversely, these same diseases are less common in countries where meat, dairy, fat and processed foods are rarely, if ever, consumed. Here are some of the comments of people following the "Peace Diet" principles, who have seen their inflammatory disease improved:

> *"I had . . . ulcerative colitis and . . . autoimmune disease and for me, it affected my . . . joints and so I was in constant pain. Now my ulcerative colitis is gone and I don't have pain anymore."* Kathy P.

> *"I had myasthenia gravis - an autoimmune disease which is like muscular dystrophy and is sort of incurable. After the program I started feeling better and when I went . . . for a checkup, the autoimmune numbers were all normal. Now I'm in remission and I don't even take medicine for that and at one point, when the condition was really bad, I was taking 24 pills a day."* Joanne G

Why the Peace Diet Cuts Inflammation and Pain

Let's look at the mechanism of the inflammatory processes. There are two main categories of factors that influence inflammation: The first is what I would call "triggering" factors, those things that cause the inflammation process to kick into gear. Some examples or triggering factors are injury, allergens, toxins, proteins, infections, and any other such insult to the body. The second main category of factors is what I call "promoting" factors -- that is, those factors causing the exacerbation and continuation of the inflammation.

Factors That Trigger Inflammation

One of the ways the Peace Diet helps to reduce inflammation is by reducing the body's load of these triggering factors from the environment. Environmental inflammatory agents are covered in greater detail in the section in this book on four of the eight enhancements to the Peace Diet. While much of inflammation may be triggered by non-dietary factors, probably the most common triggering factor in diet that we all face is allergens, whether the allergic reaction is caused by toxins, chemicals, or simply allergenic proteins found in food.

In terms of the food you eat, the Peace Diet helps to reduce inflammation because it eliminates processed food, food with toxic or irritating chemicals, dairy protein, and other proteins.[23] This reduces the body's exposure to triggering factors that might be causing long-term inflammatory problems to persist and be difficult to resolve.

For example, a lot of foods may have residual amounts of fertilizer, pesticides or herbicides on them from farming practices. Everyone should know up front that these chemicals will be in much greater concentrations in animals (including birds and fish). This is because chemicals will bio-concentrate in the creatures from the accumulated toxins that they have consumed over their lifetime. Eliminating animal products is one way that the Peace Diet helps to minimize inflammation.

Animal products also carry another category of little-known inflammatory agents that can cause inflammation without you knowing about it. Researchers have found that consuming animal products such as meat, chicken, turkey and cheese can trigger an immune response apparently through stimulating immune regulators known as "Toll Like Receptors" or TLR's. They found that this was related to the bacterial count in the animal products which can be as high as 100 million per quarter pound of meat - even if it is not spoiled. What they also found was that cooking did not prevent the inflammatory response. They concluded that the endotoxins from the bacteria were triggering the inflammation and that these endotoxins were resistant to heat and acid exposure. So, this is another reason why avoiding meat and diary helps bring peace to the inflammation battlefield in our bodies.

In terms of plant-based foods, it is important to wash vegetables, especially if they are not organic because of the chemicals that may be on them. It is also important to avoid artificial ingredients that may have been added or bio-engineered into the foods.

For example, it is important to avoid the use of hydrogenated oils of any kind. The reason for this is that the process of hydrogenation of oils creates unnatural fats known as "trans fats." The problem with eating these kinds of fats is that the body does not know what to do with these artificial fats. The result is that they are identified as foreign substances and inflammation results.

Genetically modified foods also known as Genetically Modified Organisms (GMO) are also a potential problem. Because of the way these kinds of food are bio-engineered - basically by putting imprecise sections of DNA from different organism's together - and hoping for a desirable result, there is no way to tell if they may have components that cause inflammation. For all we know, we may be producing genetically modified organisms that appear foreign or make substances that appear foreign to our bodies. This could trigger an immune response that causes inflammation, with results that we just have not studied long enough.

There is evidence that the deadly eosinophilia-myalgia syndrome associated with GMO-produced L-tryptophan in the 1990's may have been caused by severe allergy to GMO-related substances. [24] Because of this, and because of documented organ damage to animals connected to the consumption of GMO foods, some scientific organizations such as the American Academy of Environmental Medicine have called for a moratorium on GMO foods until long-term studies have been done.[28]

Because of these factors, it is safest to choose organic foods because by definition, these are foods that are not genetically modified (non-GMO) and have been grown without the use of pesticides, herbicides or artificial chemicals. If non-organic foods are used, it is important to wash the foods before consuming them.

Factors that Promote Inflammation

The second main group of factors influencing inflammatory disease is what I would call "promoting factors." Two of the main types of substances include prostaglandins and cytokines. We'll describe prostaglandins first.

A familiar way to illustrate this category is to explain how aspirin works. We all know that aspirin helps to control pain. Most people are also aware that it helps you to control fever, control inflammation, and to thin the blood; these are the drug's four main actions. The way it works is that it blocks a certain class of micro-hormones known as "prostaglandins," which control inflammation, clotting, fever, and pain. Part of the problem with taking aspirin, however, is the potential side effects it can cause: if taken on an empty stomach, aspirin can create ulcers, damage the kidneys, and cause hearing loss. As benign as the drug sounds, we must be careful with its usage.   The main precursors of these inflammatory prostaglandins are omega-6 fatty acids from two basic essential fats we've already mentioned: linoleic (omega 6) and linolenic acids (omega 3). The purpose of them is to stimulate pain, inflammation, clotting, and fever, so that the body knows to begin to heal -- useful functions, but ones that can become excessive, especially with a diet too high in omega-6 fats.

Get the Effect of Aspirin without Aspirin

If you cut prostaglandins off at their origin by reducing intake of omega-6 fats, then these four effects—pain, clotting, inflammation, and fever-- are also reduced. Thus, it's possible to get the benefits of aspirin, to some extent, by limiting intake of linoleic acid, which is present in vegetable oil in various amounts. In other words, less oil means less inflammation. The guidelines of the Peace Diet advise people to reduce their intake of vegetable oil with this goal in mind. (Of all the vegetable oils, extra-virgin olive oil is the most preferable because of its low omega-6 profile.)

Related to this discussion is, of course, the need to also limit consumption of animal products, which are typically high in another omega 6 fat: arachidonic acid. The number one source of this omega-6 fat in the U.S. is chicken. When I tell that to people, it comes as an unpleasant surprise, because they've been eating more chicken as a "healthy" alternative to red meat. I'm not saying you should go back to red meat—you'll find nearly as much arachidonic acid in virtually any other flesh food. In fact, there is virtually no arachidonic acid in plant-based foods. So, in general, animal products are pro-inflammation, and unprocessed plant products will likely be anti-inflammatory.

Pathways to Inflammation

linoleic acid (omega 6 from oils) and
arachidonic acid (omega 6 from animal products)
lead to pro-inflammatory prostaglandins

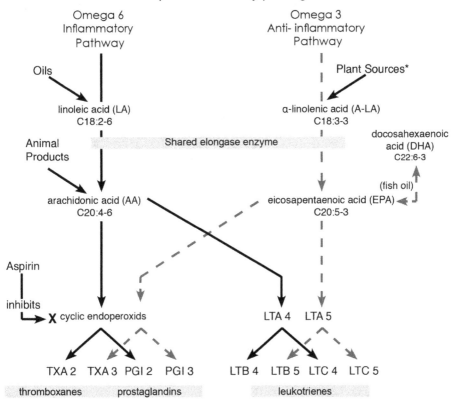

- Prostaglandins - PGI 2 Increase pain, inflammation, fever
  PGI 3 Less   "   "   "

- Leukotrienes - LTB 4, LTC 4, Increase asthma, swelling,
  sustained inflammation by attracting leukocytes
  LTB 4, LTC 5 Less asthma, swelling,
  sustained inflammation by attracting leukocytes

- Thromboxanes - TXA 2 Increase clotting (thrombosis) and blood pressure
  TXA 3   Less   "   "   "

*Some sources of α-linolenic acid are flax, chia, and hem seeds, and seaweed and greens.

Rank	Food item	Contribution to intake (%)
1	Chicken and chicken mixed dishes	26.9
2	Eggs and egg mixed dishes	17.8
3	Beef and beef mixed dishes	7.3
4	Sausage, franks, bacon, and ribs	6.7
5	Other fish and fish mixed dishes	5.8
6	Burgers	4.6
7	Cold cuts	3.3
8	Pork and pork mixed dishes	3.1
9	Mexican mixed dishes	3.1
10	Pizza	2.8
11	Turkey and turkey mixed dishes	2.7
12	Pasta and pasta dishes	2.3
13	Grain-based desserts	2

Table 4. Food sources of arachidonic acid (PFA 20:4), listed in descending order by percentages of their contribution to intake, based on data from the National Health and Nutrition Examination Survey 2005-2006

Percentage of omega 6 linoleic acid in oils

The most common sources of the omega 6 fats are vegetable oils. It is best to avoid or limit all added oils because all of them add a lot of calories (about 120 calories per tablespoon) and can raise cholesterol levels. Also be aware that many of the oils that are low in omega 6 are also high in saturated fat

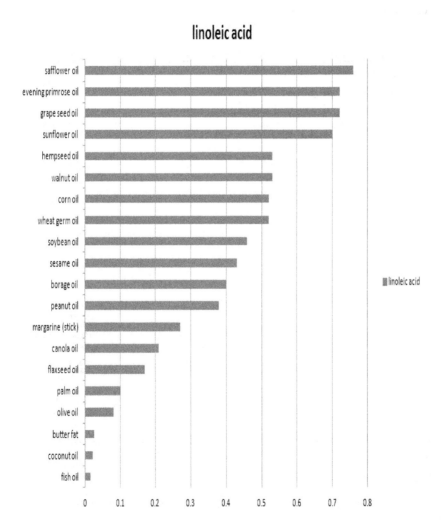

Food Sources of Total Omega 6 Fatty Acids

(Arachidonic Acid plus Linoleic Acid)

Rank	Food Item	Contribution to Intake (%)
1	Chicken and chicken mixed dishes	9.5
2	Grain-based desserts	7.4
3	Salad dressing	7.3
4	Potato/corn/other chips	6.9
5	Nuts/seeds and nut/seed mixed dishes	6.4
6	Pizza	5.3
7	Yeast breads	4.5
8	Fried white potatoes	3.5
9	Pasta and pasta dishes	3.5
10	Mexican mixed dishes	3.3
11	Mayonnaise	3.1
12	Quickbreads	3
13	Eggs and egg mixed dishes	2.9
14	Popcorn	2.6
15	Sausage, franks, bacon, and ribs	2.1

Table 2. Food sources of total omega 6 fatty acids (18:2 + 20:4), listed in descending order by percentages of their contribution to intake, based on data from the national health and nutrition examination survey 2005-2006

Saturated Fat Also Promotes Inflammation

Another important factor in inflammation is the effect of cytokines. Cytokines are a category of small proteins that have an effect on cell activity. The word "cytokine" is derived from the Latin words "cyto" which means "cell," and "kine" which is derived from the same root word as "kinetic" which means "movement." As this name implies, cytokines stimulate cellular movement of especially those cells in the immune system that contribute to inflammation. This class of inflammatory factors includes substances such as chemokines, interferons, interleukins, lymphokines, and tumor necrosis factor (TNF).

Saturated fats contribute to inflammation through a chain reaction that triggers the release of inflammatory cytokines. Saturated fats stimulate receptors known as "toll-like receptors" (TNF) that when stimulated cause the activation of nuclear factor kappa beta or NF-kB. NF-kB is a transcription factor which in turn stimulates the production of pro-inflammatory cytokines.

This inflammatory effect of saturated fat may be limited to animal fats as it appears that plant-based saturated fats such as coconut oil do not produce the same increase in inflammation. This may be because the inflammation is due to the bacterial endotoxins that may be present in animal fats but not in vegetable fats. So saturated fats should also be avoided or limited to keep inflammation in check. As for plant-based saturated fats, there may be fewer problems with inflammation, but they should be limited anyway because of the excess calories they carry and their contribution to higher cholesterol levels.

As you can see, most of the oils that are low in omega 6 fats such as linoleic acid are also high in saturated fat and vice versa. With the understanding that all food oils are lowest on the SMI scale and are likely to make weight control a little more challenging, the oils that I think is OK to use sparingly are extra-virgin olive oil and macadamia nut oil because they are low in both omega 6 and saturated fat. Canola scores well as being low in omega 6 and saturated fat, but it does contain erucic acid, which is a toxic omega 9 fatty acid. Canola comes from rapeseed, which is known to have this toxic fatty acid which can cause scarring of the heart. Even though canola as an oil has been designed to have a very low amount of erucic acid, it is still present, and much of canola is genetically modified, so I suggest using other oils.

Choose Foods That Fight Inflammation

Omega 3 fats (actually they are oils) have a calming effect on inflammation. They lead to the production of anti-inflammatory prostaglandins, leukotrienes and thromboxanes. The problem in the modern American diet (MAD) is that we consume too many oils and fats that are pro-inflammatory and not enough fats that are less inflammatory. Fish oils are famously high in the omega 3 oils called EPA (eicosapentaenoic acid) and DHA (docosahexaenoic acid). However, fish also is high in the omega 6 oil, arachidonic acid. So plant sources of omega 3 oil (alpha linolenic acid) are preferred. Some of the best plant sources of omega 3 oils are:

flax seeds, chia seeds, hemp seeds, seaweed, and leafy greens.

Inflammation promoting factors can also be reduced by choosing foods that slow the production of pro-inflammatory substances. Flavonoid-rich vegetables and fruit are very helpful in this regard. Flavonoids are not only powerful anti-oxidants. They are also strong anti-inflammatory foods as well. They inhibit an enzyme called "COX-2" or Cyclo-OXignease-2, which is the same enzyme that is responsible for the final production of prostaglandins that promote inflammation. Some foods that are high in flavonoids include:

cherries, raspberries, blueberries, blackberries, and strawberries.

Another flavonoid called quercetin helps to reduce "tumor necrosis factor" or TNF-alpha, and interleukin-8. This type of flavonoid is found in healthy amounts in apples and onions. Other flavonoid-rich foods include:

artichokes, broccoli, cucumbers, spinach, sweet potatoes, parsley, and zucchini.

Herbs that are rich in flavonoids include but are not limited to:

basil, bay leaves, cayenne pepper, ginger, mustard, nutmeg, oregano, rosemary, sage, thyme, and turmeric.

Vitamin D

Another factor to be considered in dealing with inflammatory disease is Vitamin D. Vitamin D is best known for regulating calcium and phosphorus levels in the body. A lack of Vitamin D in childhood can cause rickets, a disease of weakness in the bones. Vitamin D is actually not truly a vitamin. It is actually a steroid hormone that is produced in the skin in response to sunlight. It is called "cholecalciferol" because it has a cholesterol nucleus and because it helps in calcium absorption and regulation.

Autoimmune disease is more common in areas of the earth that have less sun exposure. Where there is less sun exposure, the classic example is multiple sclerosis: this disease is more common in far-northern and far-southern areas of the world, but uncommon near the equator. Many researchers now believe that Vitamin D inhibits some of the pro-inflammatory cytokines, the micro-substances that support inflammation.

Thus, it's important to have adequate levels of vitamin D to keep inflammation in check. The best way to do this is to get adequate--but not excessive--sunlight exposure, a factor discussed later in this book. Later, we will see that Vitamin D is also linked to the reduction in the risks of many cancers.

Blood Sugar and Inflammation

Cytokines and their effect on inflammation are also increased by high blood sugar. High blood sugar, most often associated with diabetes, is also important in the inflammatory process. When blood sugar is high, there is a much higher level of cytokines in the blood stream which causes an increase in inflammation. In clinical tests, it was shown that cytokines such as Interleukins and Tumor Necrosis Factors (TNF) were elevated.[29]   This suggests that any sudden rise in blood sugar can contribute to inflammation.

The Peace Diet helps to control inflammation in this additional way. It emphasizes whole, unprocessed plant-based foods that tend to have lower glycemic effect and higher fiber content that helps to limit the effect of cytokines and helps to bring some measure of peace to the inflammatory battles in your body.

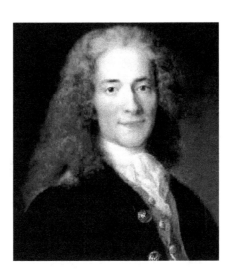

"Men fed upon carnage,
[slaughter] . . . have all an
impoisoned and acrid blood which
drives them mad in a hundred
different ways."
-VOLTAIRE (1694-1778)

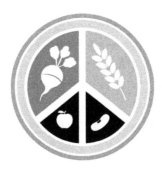

I- CONTROL BLOOD SUGAR AND DIABETES WITH A CARBOHYDRATE REVOLUTION

"When I started the program, I was taking 120 units of insulin and on the 10th day, I had to stop taking insulin altogether because my blood sugars were getting too low." Joanne G.

Another important battle in the body is the ongoing process of controlling the carbohydrates coming into your body. It is like a too much of a good thing. For example, if you have a controlled delivery of goods at a shipping harbor, it is a good thing for the users of the goods. But if, lets say, there are 10 ships trying to unload goods at the same time on a dock that is made for five ships, there would be chaos. There may be no room to stack containers while they wait for trucks to come and take them to their destinations. There may be fights over the use of fork lifts and other facilities. There may be ships backed up and blocking the harbor.

In a similar way, while carbohydrates are necessary and useful, too much of them being absorbed too quickly can cause high blood sugar and serious health problems. Over time, if you are unable to control the influx of carbohydrates and the resulting high blood sugar, you may develop diabetes.

Blood sugar levels, even among people with diabetes, are well-controlled after patients have participated in my 10-Day Program. Here are some comments from a few of those diabetics who have applied the principles of the Peace Diet and seen positive results:

> *"I was taking 75 units a day. . . In those 10 days, I got off my insulin."* Ronald T.

> *"My blood sugar dropped from two- hundred something to 81 in 10 days."* Kelly A.

> *"My blood sugar dropped to 89 and my hemoglobin test was 5.8 after over a year with no medication."* Wendy R.

Carbohydrates including starch and sugar are a natural source of fuel for your body. Your brain needs carbohydrates. It cannot function without carbohydrates, and it gets them from blood sugar. Carbohydrates are also a quick source of energy for our muscles. All carbohydrates are broken down in the digestive system and absorbed as sugar. So carbohydrates and sugars are not inherently bad for you. It is the rate of absorption that is the key.

In nature, carbohydrates from sources that are whole, plant-based foods are full of fiber and deliver carbohydrates slowly over time. When you eat foods of this kind, your body is at peace and your metabolism runs smoothly. However, if you regularly eat foods that are processed or have too much fat in them, your body has to fight to keep your blood sugar under control. If blood sugar is not controlled over the long run, the results can be catastrophic.

Sugar Clogs Capillaries - Like Cholesterol Clogs Arteries

People with chronically high blood sugar or diabetes have higher rates of heart disease, cancer, stroke, dementia, blindness, kidney failure, and amputations. These problems are caused primarily because too much sugar in the blood causes a process called "glycosylation" or the sticking of sugar to things such as proteins and enzymes. This process eventually results in an excessive amount of glocosylated proteins, and it causes unwanted deposits in the walls of capillaries. Capillaries are the tiniest blood vessels that ultimately deliver oxygen and nutrients to the cells and tissues of the body.

Just about everyone seems to know that high cholesterol causes the clogging of arteries which may lead to heart disease and strokes. In my experience, very few people know that high blood sugar causes the clogging of the tiniest capillaries. Without good circulation through capillaries, oxygen and nutrients cannot be delivered efficiently, white blood cells cannot reach infections to fight them properly, and blood cannot flow through the kidney for filtrations to occur. If this becomes severe enough, it may lead to kidney failure, poor wound healing, amputations, nerve damage, impotence, incontinence and dementia.

The Good Carbohydrate Revolution

In 2002, I wrote a book on carbohydrates called *"The Good Carbohydrate Revolution"* (Pocket Books, 2002). I so named my book because we all need to revolutionize our thinking about carbohydrates. We need to have a revolution in our way of eating in order to naturally control how fast carbohydrates enter our blood stream.

The guidelines of the Peace Diet are very helpful in controlling blood sugar levels, insulin levels, and insulin resistance. Because of this, it helps to prevent and control the more common type of diabetes, commonly known as type II diabetes.

Type II diabetes occurs when a person doesn't have good control of his or her blood sugar, usually because of the over-consumption of processed, sugary and fatty food. After eating this way for a long period of time, at some point the insulin becomes less effective. This is called "insulin resistance." The reduced effectiveness of insulin allows blood sugar to rise, and the pancreas senses this and secretes more insulin in response, causing insulin levels to rise. Contrary to popular belief, most type II diabetes is not a result of inadequate insulin production. Instead, insulin levels remain chronically high because of insulin resistance, meaning that their insulin is less effective. Having less effective insulin results in chronically high blood sugar levels which cause the body to put out more and more insulin to control the blood sugar levels.

This diet also helps with type I diabetes; however, the result is limited because in type I diabetes, the fundamental disease is not due to insulin resistance, but rather it is due to an absence of insulin. Therefore, the reversal of the insulin resistance component is not present in type I diabetes.

Four Keys to Controlling Blood Sugar

There are four keys to controlling blood sugar and reducing your need for blood sugar medication. The first key is to choose foods that are high on my SMI Food Mass Index table. This will tend to move you towards foods that will not cause a sudden rise in your blood sugar levels. It will also help to limit the number of calories you consume and increase the amount of fiber which may play an important role in slowing the rate of absorption of carbohydrates. Part of the importance of eating more fiber is that good fiber may be considered to be "prebiotics" which support healthy gut flora. Healthy gut flora is now known to play an important role in blood sugar control.

The second key is to choose carbohydrates that will have a minimal effect on your blood sugar. In my previous book, the "Good Carbohydrate Revolution" (Pocket Books, 2002), I emphasized the importance of using unprocessed food because of the effect of processing or grinding food up into a fine flour product had a dramatic effect on the effect of the food on blood sugar and insulin.

For example, in the chart below, you can see that when you turn rice into flour or potato into flour, it makes blood sugar increase even if you have the same amount of calories and grams of carbohydrate.

Blood Sugar Response to Different Forms of Carbohydrate

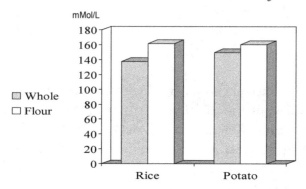

Crapo PA, Henry RR. *Am J Clin Nutr* 1988; 48:560 .

Perhaps a more important reason for using unprocessed grains is the effect of processing on insulin levels. In fact, the blood sugar would rise much higher if not for the heroic effort of the pancreas to keep the sugar down with insulin. And remember that chronically high insulin levels contribute to metabolic syndrome with weight gain, high blood pressure, and high triglycerides along with the high blood sugar. This is described in greater detail in the section on "metabolic syndrome" in this chapter.

Insulin Response to Different Forms of Carbohydrate

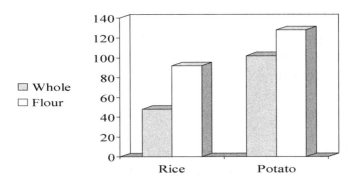

Crapo PA, Henry RR. *Am J Clin Nutr* 1988; 48:560 .

Because of the hidden rise in insulin that is required to deal with rapidly absorbed sugar, it is important to choose foods that have less of an impact on blood sugar. There is a Glycemic Index (GI) table at the back of the book to help you find foods that will have less of an impact on your blood sugar. Be careful in using the GI table, however, because the GI table will make high fat foods look better than they should. They also make some good foods such as carrots look worse than they should. The GI table is useful in comparing foods that are similar to each other such as stone ground bread compared to white bread, but be careful in comparing unlike foods. In general, using the SMI table along with the GI table will give you better guidance in finding foods that help control blood sugar.

The third key is to limit fat intake, especially saturated fat because these fats tend to block insulin receptors. This is important because the basic problem in type II diabetes is "insulin resistance" as discussed earlier. If receptors for insulin are blocked, insulin becomes less effective and insulin resistance gets worse.

The fourth key is to exercise to burn off the excess sugar. Exercise has many benefits to offer in terms of health. One of the best effects of exercise is to relieve the body of dealing with so much sugar. Exercise also contributes to an elevation in metabolic rate which helps the body to continue to burn even more sugar over time.

Metabolic Syndrome

When blood sugar is poorly controlled, another important process creates a new health problem. That is the level of insulin in the blood stream. Insulin is necessary to the body to help move sugars and amino acids from the blood stream out of the blood stream into the cells, where they can be used for energy or other important functions. This is important to keep blood sugar levels under control, so that high sugar levels don't cause damage in our bodies. However, if we chronically eat too much processed carbohydrates and fat, the system is overwhelmed and the insulin becomes less effective so that more and more insulin is needed for any meaningful control of blood sugar. If the insulin level remains high, it can cause a group of health problems together known as "metabolic syndrome." This syndrome includes overweight, high cholesterol and triglycerides, high blood pressure, and high blood sugar.

Unfortunately, the knee-jerk response to high blood sugar is to limit carbohydrates and substitute "low carb" foods such as meat, dairy and chicken instead. All too often, the condition doesn't improve and may be frustrating or worse. I've seen it time and again in my practice. There are at least five potential problems with this approach that may explain why these recommendations are not ideal.

- First, these are foods that are low on the SMI scale and high in fat, and will tend to contribute to weight gain.
- Second, because these foods are high in saturated fat, they will tend to block insulin receptors and worsen the insulin resistance.
- Third, the high fat content of these foods, especially saturated fat, increases the risk of heart disease - which is the leading cause of death in diabetes.
- Fourth, these foods will increase inflammation which may contribute to insulin resistance.
- Fifth, these foods may raise insulin levels even higher than some carbohydrates and make metabolic syndrome worse. (see chart below)

High Protein Foods Raise Insulin More than Some High Carb Foods

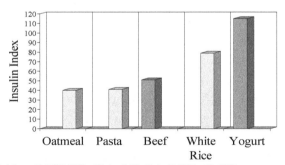

Adapted from: Holt SH, Miller JC, Am J Clin Nutr, 66:1264 - 67; 1997

Insulin and Weight Control

So what exactly is insulin, and what does it do? It is a regulatory hormone, produced in response to food after we eat it. The main purpose of insulin is to open up channels in the body's cells for sugar and amino acids to move from the blood stream into the cells where they can be used. Insulin also makes you gain weight because it is a "lipogenic" hormone, which causes the body to produce fat to store away any excess fat after a meal. In other words, after a meal or snack, insulin "stashes away" the extra calories the body doesn't need at that time as fat, a stored form of energy that can be used later.

While type I diabetes is similar in blood sugar effects, the opposite occurs in terms of insulin levels, and illustrates the important role insulin plays in weight control. Type I diabetes is actually a very different disease from type II diabetes. Type I diabetes is an autoimmune disease in which the body's own immune system destroys the cells that produce insulin. This disease, which usually starts in childhood or adolescence, is a disease in which the body produces almost no insulin. People who have type I diabetes tend to be slim because the lack of insulin makes it difficult for them to produce body fat. Probably the best known example of this is Mary Tyler Moore, a spokesperson for juvenile diabetes (type I), who has this condition and has always been slim. This is in sharp contrast to the obesity of people with type II diabetes, who gain weight so easily in part because they produce too much insulin.

The Peace Diet helps weight control not only by causing a natural decrease in calorie intake. It also is a diet that helps to control insulin levels. This makes weight control much easier because controlling insulin levels makes it more difficult for the body to produce fat.

Insulin, Cholesterol and Triglycerides

Chronically high insulin levels result in a condition known as "metabolic syndrome." This condition is a combination of high blood sugar, increased blood pressure, excess body fat around the waist, and abnormal cholesterol levels. Insulin tends to promote the build-up of fat around the waist. What's even worse is that it causes abnormal cholesterol and triglyceride levels.

Insulin tends to make things worse for heart disease by stimulating the production of cholesterol and decreasing its absorption.[30] In addition, with metabolic syndrome, triglycerides increase because insulin stimulates the production of fatty acids and triglycerides. [31]

Insulin and High Blood Pressure

Insulin also contributes to high blood pressure, and if not regulated properly, can contribute to an imbalance in cholesterol and triglycerides. Too much insulin creates "metabolic syndrome," which includes high blood sugar, high blood pressure, obesity, and high triglycerides and a bad cholesterol ratio.

In my 10-day Programs, with patients following the guidelines of the Peace Diet, participants have brought their diabetes and metabolic syndrome under much greater control. I have taken participants off as much as 80 units of insulin in 5 days, and 120 units of insulin in just 3 weeks because they had better control of their blood sugar as a result of the Program.

Of course, results vary from one person to another, but my published results show that these guidelines − despite the Peace Diet being high in carbohydrate proportion − helps most people to get their blood sugar under better control. This is consistent with populations' studies from around the world that show that diabetes is lowest in prevalence where the highest proportion of carbohydrates are consumed, such as in China and Japan. In other words, carbs aren't the "bad guy."

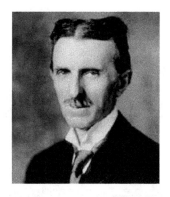

"Vegetarianism is a commendable departure from the established barbarian [meat eating] habit. That we can subsist on plant food and perform our work even to advantage is not a theory but a well-demonstrated fact. ... every effort should be made to stop the wanton, cruel slaughter of animals, which must be destructive to our morals."
-NIKOLA TESLA (1856-1943)

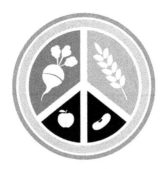

II- THE PEACE DIET AND CANCER

Diets rich in vegetables, whole grain, beans, and fruit are associated with lower rates of cancer. Did you know that the countries that eat the most meat and dairy have the highest rates of cancer - and those that consume the highest proportion of vegetables fruits and grains have the least?[32]   By choosing to eat the foods in accordance with the Peace Diet, you are helping yourself to fend off the likelihood of a cancer diagnosis in your lifetime.

Anti-Cancer Nutrients
Whole plant-based foods are all known to have anti-cancer properties. They have powerful anti-oxidants, from the more commonly-known nutrients such as the beta-carotene found in yellow and orange vegetables and fruit, to lesser known nutrients such as sulphuraphane or indoes found in cruciferous vegetables such as broccoli, epigallo-catechin gallate found in green tea, triterpenoids found in apple skins, lycopene in tomatoes, pterostilbene found in blueberries, anthocyanins found in red cabbage, and many others. The Peace Diet is also high in fiber, which is associated specifically with lower risk of stomach and colon cancer.

Vitamin C has long been considered an anti-cancer vitamin since the days of Nobel Laureate, Dr. Linus Pauling promoted it as a super-nutrient. Most people are aware that citrus fruits contain ample amounts of vitamin C in them. Vitamin C is also found in many other fruit including guava (188mg/half cup) and kiwi (140mg/2 fruit) which have more vitamin C than oranges (80mg/1 fruit) and strawberries, brussel sprouts, cantaloupe and other fruit and vegetables that have less. High dose vitamin C administered intravenously is still being researched and at least seems to help improve quality of life of cancer patients in some studies. Careful screening needs to be done because some patients and some cancers do not respond well to high-dose vitamin C according to the NCI.[33]

Vitamin D is also of great interest in the prevention of cancer because higher levels of vitamin D are associated with lower rates of certain diseases including some cancers. Blood levels in the high 50's of 25-hydroxy-Vitamin D are associated with an estimated 35% less cancer[34] including breast, colon, endometrial, kidney and ovarian cancers.

Fat Intake and Cancer

A discussion of diet and its relationship to cancer must also include a discussion of fat because high-fat diets are also associated with certain cancers all around the world. Our knowledge is not yet certain as to why this occurs, but it's possible that the countries consuming the most fat also have populations with imbalances in the hormones that are influenced by fat intake. For example, high-fat diets may cause imbalances in the male and female hormones such as estrogen which may then lead to excessive stimulation of the growth of male and female organs like the breasts and the prostate, and lead to hormone-related cancers.

Prostate Cancer Mortality vs. Fat Consumption

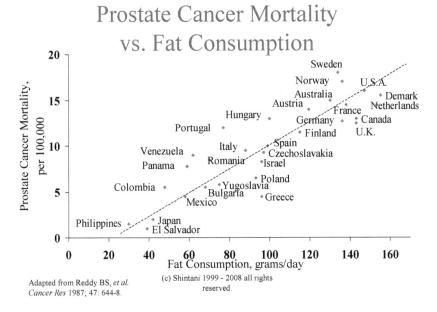

Breast Cancer Mortality in Women vs. Fat Consumption

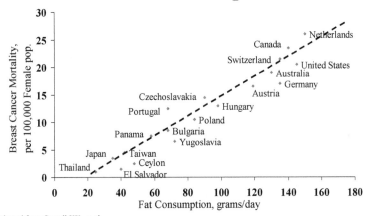

Animal Protein and Cancer

Numerous studies also correlate cancer incidence with animal protein consumption. For example, Dr. T. Colin Campbell's early research found that dairy protein (casein) was highly correlated with cancer; the more casein people ate, the higher their risk of a cancer diagnosis. In his landmark book, "The China Study," Dr. Campbell presented the connection his research had found linking animal protein intake to several cancers including breast, prostate, and colon cancer. He points out that, beyond the findings of his large-scale study of China and the regional dietary differences and cancer incidences there, other studies too had compared animal protein consumption and cancer with similar findings, thus further supporting the link between animal product intake and the protective effect of a plant-based diet. In addition, increased cancer rates are associated with high levels of methionine, an amino acid that is in much higher amounts in animal products than in plant products [35]

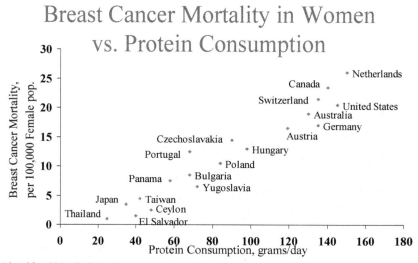

Breast Cancer Mortality in Women vs. Protein Consumption

Adapted from Dietary Fat Scatter Gram
Carroll KK, *et al.*
Cancer Res 1975; 35: 3374-83.

The Peace Diet Is Unfriendly to Cancer

In a number of ways, the Peace Diet makes the blood unfriendly to cancer cells. Not only will there be a greater presence of those cancer-preventive chemicals like those in blueberries and green tea mentioned above, there will also be an improvement in the ability of the bloodstream to attack cancer cells when they do develop. When you follow the Peace Diet carefully, factors in your blood such as insulin and IGF-1 that may support and promote the growth of cancer cells are reduced, impacting the growth of tumor cells to the point where the cancer will slow down or even start to regress. I have seen this happen on a number of occasions.

As I mentioned in the preface, my father had colon cancer when I was 6 months old. Fortunately, he survived the removal of half of his colon and a permanent colostomy. But growing up, I always wondered why there was no cure for cancer. Over the years, I heard about a variety of approaches such as the Gerson diet, which consists of organic vegetarian food. I had also heard about Hippocrates' raw-food plant-based diet as well and the Macrobiotic diet (a diet based on Oriental medicine concepts of balancing yin and yang), which for healing purposes is organic vegan and whole grain-centered. One thing these diets all had in common was that they all had examples of followers who had recovered from advanced cancer.[36]

Colon Cancer Mortality in Men vs. Fat Consumption

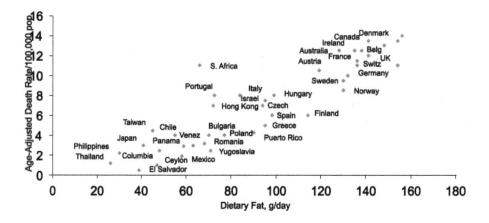

In the 1970's, laetrile was a popular, if controversial, anti-cancer substance. When I was in law school, I wrote a paper on the legal issues surrounding the use of laetrile, a substance found in apricot pits that could purportedly kill cancer cells by releasing cyanide into the cancer cell. When I looked into the Federal Register where testimonies about the laetrile controversy were kept, I found that laetrile only really worked in combination with a vegetarian diet. This got me thinking that perhaps it was the vegetarian diet, rather than the laetrile, that actually had the anti-cancer effect.

Virtually All Anti-Cancer Diets Are Plant-Based

Recalling the variety of seemingly cancer-fighting diets I was familiar with, I noticed that all these approaches had some common elements. First, all were plant-based or vegetarian. Second, they all avoided processed food and artificial chemicals. Third, they all avoided dairy foods and limited the amount of dietary protein. Putting these together, I came up with a list of the common factors I thought most effective about these diets in changing the blood environment to become unfriendly to cancer, and developed the guidelines of my Peace Diet plan from what I had surmised

1. High insulin levels in the blood stream are like fuel in a fire. All of these diets advocated low-glycemic carbohydrates and plant-based foods. A reduced intake of high glycemic foods and a replacement of them with the whole, unprocessed carbohydrates naturally low in glycemic effect, keep insulin levels steady and at low levels. Also, a diet that is relatively low (but not deficient) in protein is helpful in keeping insulin levels down because protein raises insulin levels. Beef, pork, chicken, and fish raise insulin levels more than oatmeal or even pasta.

2. Another substance similar to insulin also promotes growth of cancer cells: Insulin-like Growth Factor no.1, often called simply "IGF-1." This is a substance that is also highly correlated with a number of cancers, and it too is increased by the consumption of animal flesh.

3. Treatment for sex hormone-based cancers (such as prostate and breast) includes the administration of hormone blockers. The Peace Diet, if followed carefully, keeps fat intake low enough that excessive production of sex hormones by the body are reduced, thus helping to protect against these types of cancers.

4. Whole, unprocessed plant-based foods are loaded with not only anti-cancer substances, but also anti-inflammatory nutrients as well those that will help support the immune system, one of the body's most important defenses against cancer. A healthy immune system can

find and kill cancer cells before they get started. There are two primary white blood cell types, cytotoxic T cells and "natural killer" cells that can detect and destroy cancer cells and may play an important role in the reversal of cancer growth. A healthy diet can optimize the function of these white blood cells.

5. Fifth, the study of "epigenetics," which examines the effect of diet on gene expression, is providing interesting new research. It appears that, in places of the world with very low rates of cancer, there are dietary patterns very different from those in places of the world with much higher cancer rates. It is possible and even likely that at least one of the factors of cancer risk is the switching on of cancer-causing genes through diet. The Peace Diet reflects a food pattern consistent with lower levels of the most common cancers in the U.S.

There are undoubtedly other mechanisms yet undiscovered or not researched adequately that may contribute to the prevention, arrest and reversal of cancer. For example, the change in gut flora may have an impact on cancer, and the immune stimulation of mushrooms and other fungi may also be found to be useful.

Note: People who already have cancer should obtain the guidance of a licensed health professional to optimize their overall approach to treatment and always weigh the risks and benefits of all possible therapies when making choices.

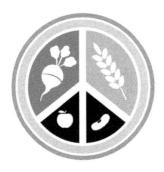

I- THE PHYSIOLOGY OF PEACE

When I changed my diet many years ago, within five days my energy level and mental alertness improved unmistakably. It was as if I were a different person. No longer was I lethargic, having difficulty getting up in the morning or tired in the afternoon. I would wake up in the morning, bright-eyed and with a clear head. And my energy would last all day. Others had a similar experience.

> *"I'm just better than healthy now. I feel great and I'm getting back to my running and exercising. . . ."* Joseph C.

> *"I feel wonderful, I have tons of energy, I can walk forever, I feel wonderful. Every day I get up and I feel happy."* Melissa T.

More importantly, I was more optimistic. My occasional feelings of depression and frustration seemed to evaporate. Others have noted similarly that their mood improves when eliminating meat from their diets.

> *"I don't eat meat because meat brings out negative qualities such as fear, anger, anxiety, aggressiveness, etc. Vegetables peacefully offer themselves to the earth when ripe, thus allowing a sublime and peaceful thought-consciousness"* Carlos Santana, Musician

Most importantly, after a few weeks, I noticed that spiritual things started happening to me. I started getting insights, and it seemed that my prayers were more effective. It was the beginning of my relationship with the Almighty. After going through this experience, I always wondered what was it about my change in diet that caused these changes to happen in me.

In this chapter, I'm going to discuss why diet can have a major effect on your thoughts, your mental attitude, your emotions and even your feeling of inner peace. This effect is supported in research on plant-based diets compared to meat-eating in terms of stress and mood. In a study published in *Nutrition Journal*, researchers found that people on a plant-based diet felt calmer than those on diets that contained flesh.[37] In another study, researchers found that vegetarians had better mood and significantly less negative emotion than omnivores, as measured by formal Depression Anxiety Stress Scale (DASS) and Profile of Mood States (POMS) questionnaires. [38]

There are at least five main categories of effects related to your diet that have something to do with your mental and emotional function. They are as follows:

Hormones
Blood sugar levels
Blood circulation
Neurotransmitters
Inflammation

Hormones

Hormones play a major role in regulating the metabolic functions of our bodies. They control our energy levels, our structure, (our skin, bones, muscle, and sexual characteristics), and to a large extent, our mood. The pituitary gland found at the base of the brain is the "master gland" and produces many hormones. It is called the "master gland" because it controls other endocrine glands by sending out stimulating hormones that signal other glands to produce more of their hormones.

Sex Hormones

Sex hormones probably have the most recognized effect on mental attitude or emotional status. Androgens and estrogens and their balance have a lot to do with why men in general are more aggressive than women, and women, more passive and nurturing. We know very well that sex hormones also affect mood. For example, when men take anabolic steroids to build muscle, they can become very aggressive and easily angered. When women have their hormones out of balance such as during premenstrual syndrome, they can become depressed or irritable. Some women become depressed, even profoundly so after giving birth. Known as post-partum depression, it is caused by an imbalance in female hormones, typically by estrogen dominance and inadequate natural progesterone.

So, how do we know that diet can affect sex hormone levels? Research shows that a high fat diet correlates to high levels of estrogens, while a low fat, plant-based diet will cause a decrease in estrogen levels.

Vegetarian Diet and Estrogens

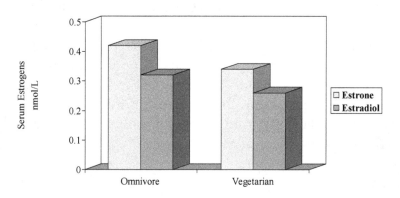

Adapted from: Goldin BR, Aldercreutz H, Gorbach SL, et al. NEJM 307(25)1982

The prevalence of meat eating may have much to do with why women today have such a high incidence of pre-menstrual syndrome. The body is really not equipped to deal with the higher levels of estrogen brought on by an artificially high-fat diet and an artificially high-animal product. Research shows, for example, that women who follow a plant-based low-fat diet have lower rates of pre-menstrual syndrome and its associated cramping or "dysmenorrheal."

Low Fat Vegetarian Diet and Dysmenorrhea

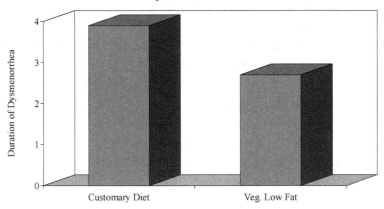

Adapted from: Barnard ND, Scialli AR, Hurlock D, et al. Obstet Gynecol 2000, 95(2) p245-50

For men, we know that androgens including anabolic steroids, can actually cause mood change as well. For example, Lyle Alzado, all-star professional football player who spoke about his anabolic steroids and said: *"I became very violent on the field and off it. I did things only crazy people do. Once a guy sideswiped my car and I beat the hell out of him."*

We know that there's a clear relationship of diet to androgen levels.[39] This excessive androgen level may be contributing to the high rates of prostate cancer in the U.S. Therefore, it makes sense to moderate excessive hormone levels by changing the diet to a more natural one of plant-based foods which are lower in fat, lower in animal products, and lower in dairy, which is often laced with artificial hormones. [40]

Thyroid Hormones

Other hormones also play a role in our health and feeling of well-being. Thyroid hormone controls our metabolic rate. If thyroid levels are inadequate, we feel lethargic, fatigued and unable to handle the day's duties. Lack of adequate "T3," the most active form of thyroid hormone, may even lead to depression. If thyroid levels are excessive, we may feel nervous and fidgety. Because of this, it is important to get all the necessary nutrients to make sure the thyroid is working properly. These include iodine, selenium, zinc, B-complex, tyrosine, and Vitamin D. It is also important to avoid toxins such as excessive radiation, chlorine, fluoride, pesticides and herbicides that could affect the function of our thyroid gland.

Adrenal Hormones

Another important group of hormones is the adrenal hormones. The adrenal gland is important to us in our stress response. When we are under stress, we produce two kinds of hormones from the adrenal gland. One type of hormone produced is adrenaline which gives us the "fight or flight" response necessary to deal with a crisis. It heightens alertness, causes pupils to dilate, and causes our heart rate to increase.

When we are under stress, our adrenal glands also produce more cortisol, which has a substantial effect on our mental, emotional and spiritual health. Too much cortisol can cause mood swings just as sex hormones can. Some call it "steroid rage" or "road rage." It can also cause weight gain.

A depletion of cortisol can also cause problems such as fatigue and depression. This can occur when people are under long-term stress that overworks the adrenal glands to a point where they burn out and become unable to produce adaptive hormones when needed. The Peace Diet helps to prevent excess hormone levels as well as keep up healthy levels of nutrients that support the adrenal glands, such as vitamin B Complex, especially pantothenic acid, vitamin C, and vitamin D. Herbs such as licorice root and ashwaganda may also be helpful.

Unnatural and Animal Hormones

Hormones from other sources may also play a role in mental calmness and spiritual peace. Considering the fact that hormones can influence our mood, we need to be aware of hormones and hormone-active that we are getting that our body does not produce. For example, some pesticides have powerful hormonal effects. Atrazine, the most commonly used pesticide, has been shown to feminize frogs even at low doses.[40]

Another source of concern is the genetic modification of food. For example, it is well known that soybeans have weak estrogenic effects. It is also known that approximately 93% of soy grown in the U.S. is genetically modified (GMO). What is not known is whether the genetic modification has somehow made the estrogenic effects stronger and or whether it has caused any new allergies or health problems. Could this be contributing to breast cancer or low sperm counts? We don't know because long-term studies have never been done on the safety and health effects of this GMO food. This is why the American Academy of Environmental Medicine has called for a moratorium on GMO foods until such safety studies have been done.[41]   This emphasizes the importance of using organic foods as much as possible because of the possibility of pesticide or herbicide contamination having a potential effect on consumers.

Another concern in regard to hormones is our exposure to animal hormones. For meat and flesh-eaters especially, this could be an important issue because animals will bio-concentrate pesticides, herbicides and any bio-active substance they consume. So, the levels of toxins or unnatural hormones in animals will tend to be higher than what might be on plants or in water because many of these substances will be trapped or held in the fat and tissues of the animals and build up over the years.

This problem may be made worse in those eating factory farm-raised animals because the animals' living conditions and slaughter processes will undoubtedly elevate stress hormones.[42] These stress hormones are ingested when a person eats these slaughtered animals. It would not be surprising if some of these hormones exerted their physiological influence and caused a person to have some of the stressful feelings of the animals that may have been induced in the slaughtering process.

Blood Sugar Levels

Another factor in controlling our mood and personal peacefulness is blood sugar levels. Blood sugar levels, especially low blood sugar levels, can cause fatigue, irritability and stress. When a person eats food that affects blood sugar levels unnaturally and causes them to swing up and down, it will affect how they feel and how they function.

If you are eating foods that are high on the glycemic index, which are largely refined carbohydrates, these foods hit the bloodstream very quickly and you'll see a spike in the blood sugar. When blood sugar spikes, the pancreas senses this rise in sugar and sends insulin into the blood stream. The insulin keeps the blood sugar level from getting too high by pushing blood sugar into the cells where the sugar can be converted into energy.

The problem comes about when you have eaten a large amount of high glycemic food and your glycemic load (glycemic index of a food times the amount of the food eaten) becomes high. What happens is that your blood insulin levels become very high because of the rush of blood sugar from high glycemic foods.

Because of this high insulin level, blood sugar is rapidly taken out of the blood stream and put into cells. Now, because high glycemic food is easily absorbed from your stomach, (especially if there is no fiber in the food to slow it down), it runs out quickly in your stomach, and there is soon no more sugar to be absorbed. Now you have a problem of high insulin levels lingering in the blood stream with no sugar coming in to replace the sugar that has been taken out of the blood stream and put into the cells. This can easily result in low blood sugar, also called "hypoglycemia."

This can cause you to feel irritable and out of sorts because your blood sugar levels are inadequate and it takes a little while before insulin levels drop and return the blood sugar back to normal. So, that's another major factor that may affect your mood. If you are eating natural foods, blood sugar will rise gradually and will drop gradually, and it will be fine.

Blood Circulation

A third factor in the control of mood and peacefulness is circulation. As you can imagine, blood flow in the brain is an important factor in how we think and feel. Capillaries, the smallest vessels in the body, have diameters that are a little over one cell wide. Their purpose is to deliver oxygen into the cells through the cell wall. They are small so the blood cells in the capillaries can touch the wall and then deliver its oxygen to where it is supposed to go. On a high fat diet, these cells begin to clump together and interrupt circulation.

For example, if blood is flowing through a capillary in the brain and a bunch of the blood cells are clumped together because of a high fat diet, gradually blood flow and oxygen delivery may be impaired. As a result, you may feel a bit out of it because you are not getting full oxygen circulation going to your brain. This effect may explain why people feel a little tired and sluggish after a high-fat lunch. The Peace Diet may be able to prevent this sluggishness because, since its fat content is quite low, the blood cells are less likely to clump together and decrease mental function. As a result, you may have a heightened sense of awareness on the Peace Diet.

Neurotransmitters

The final factor is neurotransmitters, which are the chemicals that send signals from one nerve to another and nerve signals from the brain to other parts of the body. These chemicals are stored in the tips of nerve-endings and communicate with adjoining nerves. When a nerve signal is being sent, the nerves communicate by secreting neurotransmitters at the nerve endings into the junction between the nerves. This stimulates the nerve that the nerve ending touches, and the nerve stimulated sends a signal down its nerve ending to the next nerve, and so forth. This is the way we send signals from brain cell to brain cell and nerve cell to nerve cell.

The neurotransmitter that is associated with calmness is serotonin. The more serotonin in the brain, the calmer we feel.

The precursor to serotonin is the amino acid "tryptophan." When you eat good carbohydrates, you make an amino acid called tryptophan, a precursor to serotonin, which is the neurotransmitter that makes you feel calm. So, eating good carbohydrates will actually help you to feel calmer.[43]

The flip side of this is the effect of over-consumption of animal protein. The connection between animal protein and stress has been described in several disciplines including Chinese medicine and Macrobiotics. My teacher, Michio Kushi, the founder of the Macrobiotic movement in America said:

> *Overconsumption of meat, eggs, poultry, cheese and . . . other animal quality food . . . produce general mental fatigue, . . . excitability, short temper, prevailing discontent, discrimination and prejudice, . . .*

What is it in animal products that could cause this "short temper" and "discontent"? Earlier in this chapter, I mentioned the effect of imbalance hormones that consumption of animal fat may induce. There is another factor that may affect neurotransmitters that can increase stress. When animals are slaughtered, they are placed under a great deal of stress. This causes them to produce excessive amounts of stress hormones and neurotransmitters including adrenalin. This is available in small amounts in the animal flesh. This can cumulatively lead to higher levels of stress hormones and adrenalin in the body eventually inducing feelings of stress in the person eating the flesh of a stressed animal.

Inflammation

Inflammation may also play an important role in how we feel. As we discussed in the chapter on health, the Peace Diet may be considered an anti-inflammatory diet because of the types and amounts of omega 6 fats in it. One of the key players is arachidonic acid, which is the direct pre-cursor to inflammatory prostaglandins. Arachidonic acid is generally found only in animal products.

Researchers have found in a clinical study that putting meat-eaters on a vegetarian diet actually improved their mood scores. In this study, mood scores of vegetarians were compared to those of fish-eaters and meat-eaters. The result was that the fish-eaters did slightly better than meat-eaters and the vegetarians' mood scores were significantly better.[44]

One of the mechanisms the researchers proposed was that inflammation of the brain may have played a role in the lower scores of meat and fish-eaters. They suggested that the higher arachidonic acid levels from animal products may have contributed to hither levels of inflammation in the brain. PET scan evidence already indicates that there is a correlation between arachidonic acid and inflammation of the brain in Alzheimer's disease.[45] This may explain why one of the world's top researchers in Alzheimer's disease, Dr. Rudolf Tanzi says, *"Any animal that gets old enough, will get the pathology of Alzheimers - except for herbivores."*[46] So, when you eat lots of animal products, you will likely have more arachidonic acid in your system and as a result, more inflammation in your brain than you would otherwise. This could easily contribute to your feelings of stress.

In summary, five factors that are important in terms of looking at the effect of diet in mind and mental attitude are hormones, blood sugar, blood circulation, neurotransmitters, and inflammation. There are other factors that cannot be measured as well that come into play when eating whole, unprocessed plant-based food in balance and harmony with nature. Many of the eight enhancements may play a role as well. For example, activity, exercise and sleep play a major role in your mood. Exercise is one of the best natural anti-depressant activities. Inadequate sleep results in fatigue and mood changes. Exposure to pesticides and other toxins can make you feel fatigue. Herbs can also play an important role. Energy such as true scalar energy may have a biochemically mediated anti-depressant effect.

When you follow the Peace Diet guidelines, you'll have a good chance of harmonizing all these factors to give you the best chance of optimizing your health and how you feel. In turn, it will give you the physiology to enhance calm and peaceful feelings.

The Peace Diet will give you the physiology to enhance your practice of meditation as well. A close friend of mine Sooriya Kumar from Sri Lanka established an organic farm dedicated to the teaching of arts and meditation. He named it "Mouna Farm" and explains that a vegetarian diet helps induce calmess, compassion and peace.

> *Mouna is the Sanskrit term for "inner silence." Inner silence and inner peace are one and the same. One's journey to "mouna" is a spiritual path to oneself. Once we know ourselves, we know others. Following a vegetarian diet helps induce calmness and inner peace that helps in meditation and self-knowledge. Knowing we are one and connected*

with all, compassion arises for all fellow creatures. When one feels compassion for all fellow creatures, one has reverence for them. He named it "Mouna Farm" which means "inner silence" and explains that a vegetarian diet helps induce calmness, compassion and peace. For this reason, Mouna Farm Arts and Cultural Village enjoys a vegetarian diet. www.mounafarm.org

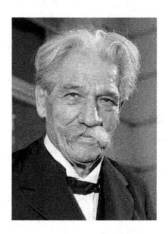

"Until he extends the circle of his compassion to all living things, man will not himself find peace."
— Albert Schweitzer (1865-1975)

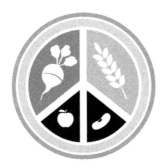

II- THE ANATOMY OF PEACE

We have an anatomy that is closer to Herbivores than to Omnivores or Carnivores. Our anatomy, especially our digestive system, gives us important clues as to what we should be eating. There are three types of mammals: carnivores, who eat almost all meat; herbivores, who eat almost all plant foods; and omnivores, who eat both. By carefully looking at the human body structure and functions, it is clear that we are supposed to eat most, if not all, of our food from plant sources.

Teeth

Teeth are a good indicator of what animals should eat. For example, carnivores like dogs and cats have sharp teeth for tearing flesh, not chewing vegetables and grains. Humans have 28 of 32 teeth clearly designed for eating grains and vegetables. We don't have a bunch of menacing sharp teeth. Our eight front teeth (the incisors), four on the top and four on the bottom, are flat. They are designed for cutting vegetables. The rear 20 teeth (10 molars and pre-molars on each jaw) are designed for grinding grains and vegetables. The remaining four "canine" teeth are possibly suitable for meat eating. In other words, seven out of eight teeth are vegetarian teeth, and possibly eight of eight.

Jaws

Another indicator that we are primarily plant-eaters is the anatomy of our jaws. Carnivores have jaw joints that are rigid and allow for up and down shearing motion so that flesh is more efficiently sliced like a pair of scissors. Omnivores such as bears and raccoons have similar jaw structures. Herbivores have loose jaw joints that allow for side-to-side motion to chew and grind plant-based foods. Human jaws are obviously of the herbivore type. Carnivores and omnivores also have their jaw joints at the same level as the molar teeth, while herbivores and humans have their jaw joints above the line of the molar teeth.

Intestine Length

Length of intestine is another important indicator of the appropriate food for a species. The length of the intestines of carnivores is short because animal-based foods have no fiber and become dry and compact. They travel slowly through the intestinal tract. The small intestines of a carnivore are three to six times the body (torso) length. Omnivores' intestinal lengths are slightly longer, four to six times the body length.

Herbivores have intestinal lengths 10 to 12 times the body length. The long intestine allows for the re-absorption of water and electrolytes of bulky plant-based stool because of the fiber content, so food can quickly travel through the intestines. Humans are more similar to herbivores than omnivores with intestinal lengths of 10 to 11 times the body length.

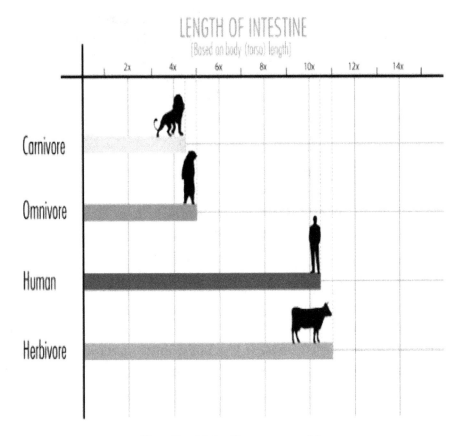

"Length of intestine compared to
torso length"

Saliva Enzyme

Amylase is a starch-digesting enzyme. The presence of this digestive enzyme, salivary amylase, in the saliva is one of the clearest indicators that humans are supposed to eat primarily plant-based food. In fact, it may mean we are supposed to eat carbohydrates in the form of starch as a primary source of calories.

This enzyme is not present in the saliva of carnivores or even most omnivores. It is found uniquely in large amounts in the saliva of humans. In fact, humans have more salivary amylase than almost all other animals, suggesting that we should be primarily carbohydrate eaters. If humans were not intended to eat plant-based food, then why is the most abundant enzyme present in the mouth an enzyme to digest complex carbohydrates?

Carbohydrates – Brain Fuel

The human brain is an obligate carbohydrate consumer. This means that our brains can't function without carbohydrates. This is another good indication that humans are supposed to eat primarily plant-based food because you don't get carbohydrates from meat, poultry or seafood. When food is abundant, the brain uses only carbohydrates as its source of energy. When there is starvation, the brain switches its metabolism so it can use fat, but it still needs at least 30% of its energy from carbohydrates. The carbohydrate requirement of the brain strongly suggests that humans are physiologically supposed to be eating primarily plant-based food.

Hands/Claws

I often tell people that if they think we are mainly meat-eaters, go into the yard and catch a bird with their bare hands like a cat could. Obviously, humans are not equipped to catch game. We don't have the claws, or the reflexes for that matter, to pounce on prey and survive. On the other hand, we have hands suitable for collecting and gathering plant foods, just like our nearest vegetarian primate relatives. Clearly, lions and tigers have the anatomical equipment such as sharp claws for catching and holding on to their prey. They also have the quick reflexes to have the speed to do so.

So, looking at the evidence of our anatomical and physiological structure, we conclude that humans are anatomically primarily herbivores. It is true that behaviorally humans were omnivores for thousands of years. But based on the evidence of our anatomy, and based on the fact that studies show humans are healthiest on a whole plant-based diet such as described by the "Peace Diet," it is clear that we should be eating primarily plant-based foods to optimize our health. This also suggests that this way of eating is one that will keep us at peace.

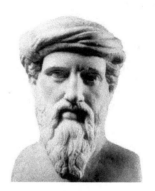

"Alas, what wickedness to swallow flesh into our own flesh, to fatten our greedy bodies by cramming in other bodies, to have one living creature fed by the death of another! ... As long as man continues to be the ruthless destroyer of lower living beings, he will never know health or peace. For as long as men massacre animals, they will kill each other."
-Pythagoras (circa 582-507 B.C.)

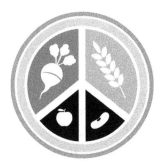

III- THE PEACE DIET: MORE THAN KARMA-FREE

Non-Killing and Peace

"In the deeper reality beyond space and time, we may all be members of one body." Sir James Jeans, Physicist (1877 - 1946)

One of the key principles in all ancient healing traditions, whether Ayurvedic, Traditional Hawaiian Healing, or Oriental Medicine, is that everything is connected. We are connected to the Earth through the food that we eat. We are connected to the atmosphere through the air that we breathe. We are connected to each other and to all living things through energy and resonance fields. If we understand this reality, then we realize that killing any sentient being, human or animal, is like killing ourselves.

Conversely, it follows that if we love others, human or animal, the love comes back to us. The law of "karma" is based on this basic assumption. It is assumed that all is connected — and good deeds will reap good fortune and bad deeds will reap bad fortune. If we ultimately achieve true health in body, mind, and spirit, we begin to feel the truth of this reality. We begin to feel the pain of others — not just humans but animals as well. When we achieve this level of health, we all see that killing animals kills our own spirit.

The great mathematician and philosopher Pythagoras said

> *For as long as man continues to be the ruthless destroyer of lower living beings, he will never know health or peace. For as long as men massacre animals, they will kill each other. Indeed, he who sows the seeds of murder and pain cannot reap joy and love.*

As previously mentioned, the concept of non-killing is one that is found in many religions and philosophies. As Pythagoras indicates, when humanity is inhumane to animals, the inhumanity somehow finds its way into the human psyche and allows humans to be inhumane to each other.

Animals are intelligent

Some whales have brains more than five times the size of a human brain. Dolphins' brains are slightly larger and orca brains are nearly twice the size of a human's. One of the most stunning videos revealing the intelligence of sea mammals is about an orca apparently attempting to communicate with a human by imitating the sound of the motor of his boat. [47]

It seems that the orca has the logic to imitate the sound of the boat - a sign of at least a fair level of intelligence. What is even more impressive is evidence that cetaceans and dolphins develop individual and unique cultures within their pods, apparently systematically taught to their descendants and carried on within the pod. By the way, an orca brain which is more than twice the size of a human brain also has more convolutions suggesting the capacity for a high level of intellect.

I'm a pet owner, and I love my little dogs. I think anyone who owns a pet knows that pets have intellect and have feelings. We all know how dogs whimper and whine when left alone or left in a cage, and express joy and enthusiasm at the return of their master. Dogs are quite intelligent and can be taught a lot of behaviors such as leading a blind person and sniffing for drugs. And what about their loyalty? Dogs are known to protect their masters from intruders, help them when they are ill or in an emergency and bark for help when help is needed.

There is also the legendary but true Japanese story of the Akita dog named "Hachiko," of which two movies have been made. Hachiko would follow his master to the train station every day and come back to wait for his return. One day, Hachiko's master died at work and never returned. Nonetheless, Hachiko waited loyally at the train station every day for years at the time his master would have arrived and did so until he died. Because dogs are so intelligent, and because they serve as companions to humans so commonly, it is unthinkable to eat a dog in the U.S.

So why is it OK to eat cow or pig? Pigs are actually considered to be more intelligent than dogs. They are said to be able to learn tricks and behaviors even more quickly than dogs. One of the best discussions of this strange dissonance is described in a book *Why We Love Dogs, Eat Pigs, and Wear Cows* by Melanie Joy, PhD. She points out that we have no problem eating pigs and cows, but if someone said that there was dog meat in our stew, most of us would be repulsed. But why?

The answer is that we find eating dog repulsive for the same reasons Hindus would find that eating "beef" or the flesh of a dead cow repulsive. It all comes down to conditioning and the shaping of our attitudes through our culture. For example, why do we call pig flesh "ham" or "pork?" Why do we call dead cow meat "beef?" Is it to protect us from the idea that this was once a living, breathing, feeling animal?

Animals feel pain

When I was in elementary school, I remember one of my teachers telling the class that he had just been to a pig slaughterhouse. He was visibly shaken when he told the story of how the pig was held down and squirmed and squealed loudly as its throat was slit. The pig did not die immediately. It struggled to escape as blood flew everywhere and kicked and screamed until it finally bled to death. It sickened him so much he never wanted to eat pork again. Imagine this happening 315,000 times per day to pigs and 114,000 times a day to cows and calves.

What's even more sickening is that in the most gruesome path of a cow to carcass to cuts of meat, the animals are supposed to be killed first but sometimes the animals are not dead. Sometimes animals are alive while they are getting skinned and their limbs chopped off.

> *On bad days dozens of animals reached his station clearly alive and conscious. Some would survive as far as the tail cutter, the belly ripper, the hide puller.*[48]

How is this not a crime?

Beyond Karma-Free Eating

The Peace Diet can also be described as "karma-free" eating. The concept of karma comes from the Hindu religion in which it is believed that good fortune today is a result of good deeds in the past — either in this life or your past life, and bad fortune is a result of some bad deeds or "karma." However, I don't believe we are ever "free" of karma. There is good karma and bad karma, and we are always under it influence. This is similar to the concept in the Judeo-Christian religion (Galatians 6:7); paraphrased, it is "*As ye sow, so shall ye reap.*"

As we kill animals, we kill ourselves

Sometimes I start my lectures by asking the question, "What is the leading cause of death of animals?" The answer is "humans" because we slaughter animals by the billions. Then I ask, "What is the leading cause of death of humans?" And the answer is "animals" because we eat them. What do I mean by this? The consumption of animals in excess is related to the top three causes of death, heart disease, cancer, and stroke. In addition, the consumption of animal products contributes to diabetes and Alzheimer's disease, among many other diseases and health conditions. It seems that the law of "karma" or some form of universal justice is operating whether we are aware of it or not and whether we like it or not.

The Peace Diet, in which no sentient beings are killed for food, does not incur the "karmic debt" of having caused a painful death of an animal. It also does not support the commerce that perpetrated the horrendous atrocities committed against billions of animals each year. In following the Peace Diet, you are free from the concern that somehow, in some way, the laws of "karma" will come around to you and eat you as you have eaten others. Perhaps more importantly, by living a life of "non-killing" and non-violence, you will lead a more peaceful life.

The Peace Diet & the Environment

Karma also manifests in our actions and how it affects our world – not just animals. Killing meat not only kills animals; it destroys the environment as well. The meat industry harms the environment in massive ways, from wasting resources as animals raised for food eat enough grain to feed the world, to a waste of fuel, to the pollution caused by their waste matter, and much more.

The Peace Diet Contributes to Better Air Quality

According to the U.N.'s Food and Agriculture Organization, meat production accounts for 18% of annual greenhouse-gas emissions. The Peace Diet avoids meat consumption and thus does not contribute to the mounting problem of greenhouse gasses.

The Peace Diet Won't Further Climate Change

Millions of acres of rain forest are cut down each year to make way for cattle ranchers and suppliers of animal feed, destroying one of the world's great "carbon sinks" and further hastening climate change. To combat the worst effects of climate change, a recent United Nations report concluded that we need a global shift toward a vegan diet.

The Peace Diet Doesn't Pollute the Water

To grow one pound of grain requires about 25 gallons of water. To produce one pound of beef requires an astonishing 390 gallons of water. Further, animal agriculture contaminates water supplies with pesticides, herbicides, and fertilizers used to grow food for the animals, polluting rivers and streams.

The Peace Diet Protects the Land

Livestock grazing erodes the topsoil and dries out the land, leading to desertification and preventing the land from sustaining plant growth. Also, it takes far more land to raise animals than to grow enough plants to feed the same number of people directly.

The Peace Diet Conserves Fossil Fuels

The production of meat, eggs, and dairy products utilizes a significant amount of fossil fuels to transport animal feed and animals as well as to run machinery on the factory farms where animals are raised.

The Peace Diet Can Help to Save the Earth

One way to help save the environment is clearly to eat a plant-based diet. Says John Robbins, author of "Diet for a New America" and "The Food Revolution":

> *It is increasingly obvious that environmentally sustainable solutions to world hunger can only emerge as people eat more plant foods and fewer animal products. To me it is deeply moving that the same food choices that give us the best chance to eliminate world hunger are also those that take the least toll on the environment, contribute the most to our long-term health, are the safest, and are also, far and away, the most compassionate towards our fellow creatures.*[49]

The Peace Diet and Feeding the World

There is enough food on this planet to feed the entire human population. Research suggests that we can feed up to 10 billion people on a plant-based diet.[50]   So, why do more than a billion people go hungry? Blame this sad reality largely on our meat-based diet. Rather than feeding those who are starving, we fatten up animals with huge amounts of grain, soybeans, and corn. If we used the crops to feed humans instead, we could easily feed everyone on the planet with healthy and affordable vegetarian foods.

The United Nations confirms this. They estimated that the 1992 food supply could have fed about 6.3 billion people on a purely vegetarian diet, 4.2 billion people on an 85% vegetarian diet, or 3.2 billion people on a 75% vegetarian diet.

Fortunately, some countries have begun to take steps in this direction. In Belgium, the Flemish city of Ghent has designated every Thursday as "Veggiedag" – Veggie Day – encouraging meat-free meals to be served in schools and public buildings, and, to encourage a vegetarian diet, promoting vegetarian eateries and offering advice on how to follow a herbivorous diet.

"He who has no ear to listen to the way is ignorant like an ox. He grows in size but not in wisdom"

Ancient Buddhist Saying

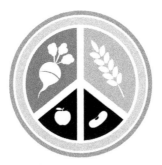

IV- ANCIENT WISDOM FOR MODERN HEALTH AND PEACE

The connection between diet, health, and peace comes from a combination of ancient wisdom and modern science. I believe in an approach that is "evidence based." The "evidence" that I use is beyond just science because the reality is that science doesn't provide all the answers. You may get knowledge from science but not wisdom. Knowledge comes from scientists and researchers, and wisdom comes from elders and prayer.

The Peace Diet is based in part on modern science and ancient wisdom found throughout human history. Numerous ancient writings indicate that a plant-based diet is ideal for humans and is conducive to spiritual development and peace. Throughout this book are quotations from notable sources and people who support a plant-based diet for ethical, health, or spiritual reasons.

Old Testament

The Old Testament, relied on by both Christianity and the Jewish faith, describes God's creation of the world and of humankind. In the book of Genesis, it says,

And behold I have given you every herb bearing seed which is upon all the face of the earth and every tree in which the fruit of the tree yielding seed it shall be for food. Genesis 1:29

Clearly, the original diet of the Almighty Father is all plant-based or "vegan," in other words, free of any animal products. In Genesis 9:4-5 God says, *"And your life will I seek at the hand of every creature that you slay…"* a direct edict from God that we should not be killing creatures of the Earth.

So from the very beginning of the rules of the Judeo-Christian Biblical book of Genesis, a series of scriptures talks about a plant-based diet as the original way of eating that God intended. Why then do so many folks feel justified eating animals? What I frequently hear is that animals don't have souls, only humans do. But the Bible itself clearly states that animals *do* indeed possess a soul. In Genesis 1:30, it states:

And to every beast of the earth and to every fowl of the air and to everything that creeps on the earth, wherein there is a living soul I have given every green herb as meat …

Note that at least some translations of the Bible say "soul," [46] which suggests that there is a living SOUL in every beast, fowl, and thing that creeps on the Earth. In other words, if the Bible may be acknowledging that animals have souls, we should not be taking the life of creatures because they have a soul.

Certainly, in the Bible, there is permission to eat flesh that comes after the flood - a time when vegetation had been wiped out by the flood. However, it doesn't diminish the fact that a plant-based diet was the original diet sanctioned for humans, and it appears that the longevity of humans decreased thereafter.

The Book of Daniel

The superiority of a plant-based diet is described in the book of Daniel, Chapter 1. Daniel was chosen along with three of his friends by King Nebuchadnezzar to be among his many advisors. When the King required all his prospective advisors to eat "the King's meat," Daniel requested that he and his friends be given vegetables and water instead. After 10 days of eating this way, he and his friends were described to be healthier than all the others. Later, the king judged them to be "ten times smarter" than the other advisors.[51]

Later, the king had a dream that he couldn't remember and he asked his advisors if they could tell him what the dream was and interpret its meaning. The king was enraged when none of them could and was about to execute them all for being incompetent. Daniel saved the day when he was able, after prayers, to tell the king what his dream was. He saved himself and his fellow advisors from execution when he was able to have a spiritual connection to the Lord who gave him the ability to describe and interpret the King's dreams.[52]

Essene Gospel of Peace

Around the time of Jesus, a sect of Judaism called the Essenes existed. Their existence was brought to life by the discovery of the "Dead Sea Scrolls." One of the translations resulted in a volume called the "Essene Gospel of Peace." In this document, it is clear that the Essenes valued a plant-based diet and were strongly against eating flesh.

> *Thou shalt not kill, for life is given to all by God, and that which God has given, let not man take away. For I tell you truly, from one Mother proceeds all that lives upon the earth. Therefore, he who kills, kills his brother. And from him will the Earthly Mother turn away, and will pluck from him her quickening breasts. And he will be shunned by her angels, and Satan will have his dwelling in his body. And the flesh of slain beasts in his body will become his own tomb. For I tell you truly, he who kills, kills himself, and whoso eats the flesh of slain beasts, eats of the body of death.* [53]

The New Testament

The New Testament in the Christian Bible does not contain much discussion about diet. There is, however, some mention of fish and fishermen. This presents a controversy as to whether or not people should be eating the original diet described in Genesis 1:29 or whether their diet should include flesh including fish. At least some biblical scholars, however, believe that Jesus followed the practices of the Essenes, and was therefore vegetarian and that John the Baptist, because of the area in which he was born, was an Essene. [54]

Some believe Paul the apostle, being from the Nazarene sect, may have been vegetarian because the Nazerenes followed Essene principles. There are also writings that suggest that the apostle Mark was vegetarian. A noted writer of an early Christian church, Clement of Alexandria in the 2nd and 3rd century said, *"It is far better to be happy than to have bodies that act as graveyard for animals, accordingly the apostle Mark partook of seeds of nuts and vegetables without flesh."*

Bread & FRUIT

One of the miracles of Jesus is the multiplying of the loaves of bread and fish to serve thousands of people. Interestingly, it may actually have been bread and FRUIT, rather than fish. There is evidence that is described in a book titled "Food for the Spirit" by Steven Rosen in which he mentioned that before the 4th century in the earlier writings of Bible manuscripts, this miracle was not bread and fish, but bread and fruit, and only in the later editions of the New Testament is fish mentioned.[56]

Christian Leaders

Going forward throughout Christianity other writings support a plant-based diet. St. John Chrysostom, who lived in the later part of the 4th century and the early part of the 5th century and was one of the earliest writers about Christianity, wrote that, *"With the Christian leaders practice abstinence from the flesh of animals to subdue our bodies the unnatural eating of flesh meat is polluting."*[57]

In later Christian sects numerous Christian leaders have supported following plant-based diets. One of the most famous was Ellen White, who was one of the founders of the Seventh-day Adventist church, which openly advocates a vegetarian diet and has many publications about a plant-based diet. Methodist

John Wesley, the founder of the Methodist church, was also known to be vegetarian. Sylvester Graham, famous for Graham crackers and one of the most famous Presbyterian Ministers, was a strong proponent of a meatless way of eating.

There are also physicians who have been strong Christian advocates of a plant-based diet. Probably the most famous of these is Dr. John Harvey Kellogg, the inventor of the corn flake. He was the medical director of one of the most successful sanitariums in American history, where they used vegetarian diet and other lifestyle and non-invasive modalities as a primary therapy for their patients. He says,

> *When we eat vegetarian foods, we needn't worry about what kind of disease our food died from; this makes a joyful meal!* -- John Harvey Kellogg, M.D.

Hindu Religion

In Hinduism most of the practitioners are vegetarian and numerous Vedic injunctions oppose meat eating. For example, one says,

> *"You must not use your God-given body in killing God's creature..."* Another Veda says, *"By not killing any living being one becomes fit for salvation,"* while another Veda says that, *"He who desires to augment his own flesh by eating the flesh of other creatures lives in misery in whatever species he may take his birth."*[58]

In the tradition of Hindu belief in reincarnation in the ancient Vedic leader church, two of the biggest writings were the Marabarata and Ramayana. The Ramayana informs us that elevated souls shun meat eating and violence, again exhorting people to non-violence, a principle advanced by one of the most famous vegetarians, Mahatma Gandhi. The doctrine found in the hymns in the ancient Hindu tradition was advanced by the great Mahatma Gandhi, non-injury to sentient beings. This was enunciated in the Vedas, the ancient Sanskrit scriptures and hymns as a means of non-violence or again, non-injury to sentient beings.

Zoroaster

The idea of animal products being undesirable is also described in Zoroastrianism, a sect that flourished in ancient Persia.[59]   In one of this religion's earlier legends in Ferdowsi's epic the *Shahnameh*, It is said that in the region's early days, people were vegetarian. *"Foods then were few, yet people did not kill to eat But lived on the earth's produce of vegetal."*

Meat-eating was considered an evil habit as indicated by the role of Ahriman, the devil incarnate. Ahriman used meat-eating to gain favor with Zahhak, the King, and eventually took control of him by stimulating his carnal lust for blood and flesh.

Sikhism

Sikhism, while not strictly known as a vegetarian belief system, acknowledges the importance of avoiding meat in spiritual enhancement. It was founded by Guru Nanach in the 1400s and 1500s. It is to some extent a religion born of a mix of Hindu and Islamic principles, but a number of the gurus have adopted the traditional Hindu style of vegetarian eating. Guru Nanach considered meat-eating improper, especially for those who are trying to meditate, suggesting that meat-eating to some extent blocks spiritual development and only vegetarian food is allowed at their temples.[60]

Jainism

Jainism, another eastern religion found in India, has as its cardinal teaching "ahimsa" — the Indian concept of non-violence to living things. They were strict vegetarians, and they were famous in India for putting together animal hospitals. It was a Jain or Jain monk Hiravijaya-Suri who persuaded the Muslim emperor Akbar to prohibit killing of animals. Later, Emperor Akbar became himself vegetarian, although there were debates whether he was a strict vegetarian. Nonetheless, Jainism promoted the vegetarian way of eating and Emperor Akbar was supportive. [61]

Buddhism

In Buddhism, the Gautama prince or Buddha himself, was known for compassion and his love for animals. There's an ancient poem that was said to be the only text that was directly written by Buddha himself, and it says,

> *"Creatures without feet have my love,*
> *And likewise those that have two feet,*
> *And those that have four feet I love,*
> *And those, too, that have many feet. . . .*
> *Let creatures all, all things that live,*
> *All beings of whatever kind,*
> *See nothing that will bode them ill!*
> *May naught of evil come to them!"*[62]

In other words, Buddha himself is against the killing of animals and of course that would imply killing of animals for food. In Buddhism, there is a sutra that says, "The eating of meat extinguishes the seed of great compassion..." also implying that eating of meat actually arrests or somehow diminishes our spiritual growth.

This is a common theme. It seems that many wise and holy people in various religions experienced the effects of a plant-based diet elevating the spirit. They also noticed that eating meat blocks spiritual development. In the Buddhist tradition that spread throughout Asia, the concept was advanced by committed vegetarian political leaders like the great emperor Ashoka of India. He stated,

> *The greatest progress of righteousness among men comes from the exhortation in favor of non injury to life and abstention of killing beings...* [63]

This statement actually pertains also to animals. He is talking about not just health but also that meat eating in attempt to develop spiritual development becomes a problem.

Another sutra called the Lankavatara states:

> *Meat-eating in any form, in any manner, in any place, is unconditionally and one and for all prohibited. . . . Meat eating I do not permit it for any one I will not permit . . .*[61] *This is a description of Buddha that suggests that it is a direct quote from Mahayana about what Buddha had taught. Another sutra says, "How can a seeker who hopes to be a deliverer of others himself be living in the flesh of other beings. . .*[64]

So, Buddhism clearly supported plant-based diets. Many people say that Quan Yin is to Buddhism as St. Francis of Assisi is to

Christianity. Quan Yin is the embodiment of mercy and compassion in Buddhism and is the quintessential "bodhisattva" or person who is able to ascend to nirvana but remains on earth to save others. Supreme Master Ching Hai, founder of the "Quan Yin Method" is a strong advocate of vegan eating as part of the pathway to enlightenment. She states in her introductory booklet, "The Key of Immediate Enlightenment[65],"

> *So in a very real sense, the keeping of a vegetarian diet is a gift which we give to ourselves. We feel better, the quality of our lives improves as the heaviness of our karmic indebtedness diminishes, and we are offered entrance into new subtle and heavenly realms of inner experience.[66]*

As part of the mission of this group devoted to the teachings of Quan Yin, a worldwide chain of restaurants called "Loving Hut" serving vegan food may be found around the world.

In Zen Buddhism in Japan, they talk about the achievement of Samadhi or the inner state of peace. They believe that one of the most important aspects of reaching this state of being is following "shojin ryori" or spiritual development meals. These meals follow the precept of "non-killing" and thus include no animal products. The fact that this is a manner of eating to develop spirit and that it is vegan suggests that even in the Japanese Buddhist tradition, eating animals was seen to be something that would inhibit the development of the spirit. [25] The foods consisted of rice, vegetables, beans or tofu, and seasonal fruit. The meals were simple and balanced for taste and nutrition. Those who would prepare "shojin ryori" are taught to "*pour the spirit of heaven and earth into each dish.*"[67]

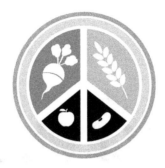

V- THE PEACE DIET PLATE

It is no coincidence that the "Peace Plate" that I have put together looks like the "Peace Sign," universally used to represent peace and a familiar sign commonly used in the peace movement. To some extent, the Peace Plate that I have put together is similar to the "My Plate" diagram put out in 2011 by the department of human services under President Obama's administration. The Peace Plate, however, is designed as a guide for eating for optimal health and *spiritual development*. Thus, this "Peace Plate" is designed to encourage a way of eating that supports the health and peace of ourselves and our world.

I made this "Peace Plate" intentionally quite simple so it would be memorable and easy to follow. As described in the introduction, it is a circle, divided down the center vertically and with dividing lines starting at the center of the vertical line and angling downwards symmetrically on each side starting at the center of the circle and ending at the edge of the circle.

On the left side, or half of the plate, the larger top portion would be vegetables, covering about 30 to 35% of the plate and a smaller portion at the bottom would be for fruit at about 15% to 20%. On the right hand side of the plate, the "Peace Plate" has Whole Grain at the top in the larger section of the right half of the diagram representing 30 to 35% of the plate, and Beans & Legumes at the bottom for 15-20% of the circle.

Dr. Shintani's
PEACE PLATE

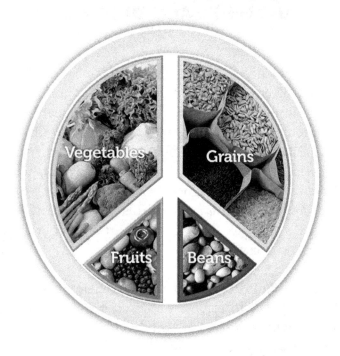

Vegetables

Vegetables are a major part of the Peace Diet as they contain the most micronutrients that are essential for optimal health. Study after study shows the consumption of vegetables to be associated with longer life and lower risk of diseases. For instance, the brassica family of vegetables has powerful anti-cancer nutrients, such as sulfuraphane. The orange and yellow vegetables, carrots, squashes, pumpkins and sweet potatoes for example, are loaded with carotenoids such as beta carotene, which is also known to have anti-cancer properties. White vegetables like onions and garlic have allicin in them and cabbages have anthocyanins which are powerful anti-inflammatory and anti-oxidant compounds.

Vegetables of all colors should represent 30 to 35% of the whole diet, both raw and cooked.

We should eat vegetables from all the various parts of the plant.

Sprout vegetables:
Alfalfa sprouts, mung bean sprouts, brussels sprouts
Root vegetables:
Carrots, beets, burdock, lotus, ginger, turmeric
Bulb vegetables:
Onion, garlic
Stem vegetables:
Celery, kohlrabi, rhubarb
Stem shoots:
Asparagus, bamboo shoots
Leafy vegetables:
Cabbage, lettuce, kale, collard greens, watercress, bok choy, choi sum, beet greens, dandelion greens, sea vegetables,

<u>Flower Buds:</u>
Broccoli, cauliflower,
<u>Fruit vegetables:</u>
(Botanically fruit but used as vegetables) tomato, squash, Pumpkin, zucchini, peppers, cucumber, avocado
<u>Pod vegetables:</u>
(overlaps with legumes) green beans, peas, snow peas, string beans

Follow the Rainbow

The benefits of vegetables and fruits come from the rainbow of colors they comprise, with each color having different healing properties.[68]

*But the wisdom that comes from
heaven is first of all pure; then
peace-loving . . .*
James 3:17

GREEN in vegetables and fruits contains phytochemicals to keep you healthy. For example, the carotenoids *lutein* and *zeaxanthin* that are found in spinach, collards, kale and broccoli have strong antioxidant properties that help protect your eyes by keeping your retina strong. Green also reduces the risk of some cancers, and promotes strong bones and teeth. And green provides antioxidants to help with memory retention and boost brain power.

The following are good sources:

Fruits

Avocadoes
Green apples
Green grapes
Limes
Honeydew
Kiwifruit

Vegetables

Green peas
Artichokes
Arugula
Asparagus
Broccoflower
Broccoli
Broccoli rabe
Brussels sprouts
Spinach
Chinese cabbage
Green beans
Celery
Cucumbers

Lettuce
Green onions
Watercress
Peas
Green peppers
Snow peas
Okra
Sugar snap peas
Zucchin
Endive
Kale
Leafy Greens
Leeks

RED AND PINK in fruits and vegetables contains the antioxidant *lycopene*. Lycopene reduces the risk of some cancers, protects against heart disease and against urinary tract infections. Lycopene also helps improve memory and protects the brain from disease

The following are good sources:

Fruits

Tomatoes
Red apples
Blood oranges
Cherries
Watermelon
Cranberries
Red grapes
Goji

Berries
Pink/red grapefruit
Red pears
Pomegranates
Raspberries
Strawberries
Guava
Papaya

Vegetables

Beets
Radishes
Radicchio
Red Onions
Red potatoes
Rhubarb

YELLOW/ORANGE Orange pigments in food come from the antioxidant beta-carotene and the whole family of carotenoids which helps vision, the heart, and the immune system and reduces the risk of cancer. Bright yellows are also high in essential vitamins and flavonoids. Pineapple, for example, is replete with Vitamin C, manganese and the natural enzyme, bromelain, a digestive aid.

The following are good sources:

Fruits

Yellow apples
Apricots
Cantaloupe
Yellow figs
Grapefruit
Golden kiwifruit
Lemons
Mangoes
Nectarines
Oranges
Papayas
Peaches
Yellow pears
Persimmons
Pineapples
Tangerines
Yellow watermelon

Vegetables

Yellow Beets
Carrots
Butternut Squash
Yellow Peppers
Pumpkin
Yellow Summer
Squash
Sweet Corn
Sweet Potatoes
Yellow Tomatoes
Yellow Winter Squash

WHITE/TAN vegetables from the onion family contain the phytochemical *allicin* which has natural antibacterial and antimicrobial properties, increases the body's ability to fight infections, and helps lower cholesterol and blood pressure.

The following are good sources:

Fruits	Vegetables
Dates	Cauliflower
Brown pears	Garlic
	Ginger
	Jerusalem artichokes
	Jicama
	Kohlrabi
	Mushrooms
	Onions
	Parsnips
	Potatoes
	Shallots
	Turnips
	White corn

BLUE/PURPLE vegetables are loaded with flavonoids and valuable phytochemicals. Purple foods may be especially beneficial for the brain. *Anthocyanins*, the phytochemical that gives foods their purple color, is believed to possibly stave off memory loss and to improve learning ability, memory, and coordination

Fruits
    Açai (ah-sigh-eee)
    Blackberries
    Blueberries
    Concord Grapes
    Dried Plums
    Elderberries
    Grape Juice
    Purple figs
    Purple grapes
    Plums
    Raisins

Vegetables
    Black Olives
    Olives (preferably sun-dried)
    Purple Cabbage
    Eggplant (Aubergine)
    Purple Peppers
    Purple Potatoes

Get Your Calcium from Vegetables

I would emphasize that a portion of the vegetables be high-calcium vegetables such as dark leafy greens and sea-vegetables. A lot of people think that the only way to get enough calcium is by consuming dairy products. The truth is that most of the world gets adequate amounts of calcium without consuming dairy foods.

After all, where does the cow get calcium? It's not drinking milk. It's eating greens. And so I think getting calcium from dairy is really a secondary source. You should really get your calcium from a direct source which is high-calcium greens, dark leafy greens such as broccoli, kale, collard and watercress and choi-sum (Chinese broccoli), as well as sea vegetables such as hijiki, wakame, kombu, etc. and black strap molasses, tofu, and almonds.

The Evolving Calcium Table

Comparison of calcium from one cup of selected foods.[a]
Calcium tables should display absorption and calcium loss.

Food	Portion 1 cup (gm)	Calcium (mg)	Fraction Absorbed[b]	Estimated Absorption (mg)	Loss Due to Protein
Kelp *(konbu)*	144	242	0.59[c]	142.8	
Wakame *(seaweed)*	144	216	0.59[c]	127.4	
Watercress	144	169	0.67	113.2	
Kale *(from frozen)*	130	178	0.588	104.7	
Turnip Greens	144	198	0.516	102.2	
2% Milk	244	297	0.321	95.3[d]	Significant[d]
Broccoli	155	178	0.526	93.6	
Tofu	126	258	0.310	80.0[d]	Significant[d]
Mustard Greens	144	128	0.578	74.0	
Spinach	180	244	0.051	12.4[e]	

In fact, the countries that consume the most dairy have the highest rates of osteoporosis.

Dairy vs. Osteoporosis

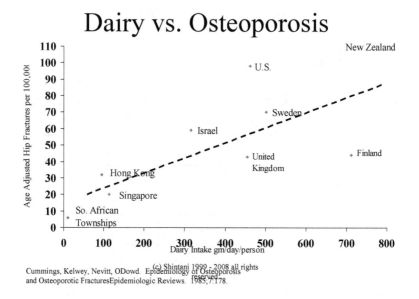

Cummings, Kelwey, Nevitt, ODowd. Epidemiology of Osteoporosis and Osteoporotic FracturesEpidemiologic Reviews. 1985, 7:178.

This high rate may be accounted for in part because countries that consume a lot of dairy also consume lots of meat and therefore a lot of protein - much more than necessary. Protein acidifies the blood, and the body's natural response is to neutralize the acid with calcium from the bones in the same way that calcium carbonate (active ingredient in Tums®) neutralizes acid stomach. As a result these populations, start losing calcium and start losing bone density. Studies show that by age 65 the average meat-eater has twice the bone loss of vegetarians.

The American Journal of Clinical Nutrition, March 1983 reported the results of the largest study of bone density in the U.S. Researchers at Michigan State and other major universities found that, by the age of 65:

Male vegetarians had an average measurable bone loss of 3%. Male meat-eaters had an average measurable bone loss of 7%.

Female vegetarians had an average measurable bone loss 18%. Female meat-eaters had an average measurable bone loss of 35%.[69]

Also, dairy products are a very poor source of calcium, since this form of calcium is very poorly absorbed (less than 1/3) by the human body.

Grains

On the right hand side of the plate, the large upper section is "whole grain" and is approximately 30 to 35% of the circle. Whole grains represent a large part of the Peace Diet, partly because it has been the main staple for the most successful civilizations throughout history. In Europe they ate wheat, rye and barley. In Asia they ate rice, wheat and millet. In the Americas they ate maize, amaranth, and quinoa. In Africa, they ate barley, sorghum and millet. In this section, you could also include other starchy staples such as sweet potato, taro, cassava, yams, and other similar root vegetables.

Nutritionally, whole grains are an important source of good carbohydrates, vitamin B complex, vitamin E, good quality fiber, and some protein. It usually comes as a surprise to most people that grains have good quality protein in them. For example, brown rice is approximately 8.4% protein, 6.7% fat, and 84.9% carbohydrate. A cup of brown rice provides about 4 1/2 g of protein. What surprises people even more is that even white rice provides about 4.4 g of protein per cup. For a more complete discussion about the adequacy of protein in the Peace Diet, please see the discussion about protein in this chapter.

In this Whole Grain section, it is very important to emphasize that you should use "unprocessed" whole grain. Be careful when buying "whole grain bread" as it is commercially processed into a finely ground-up flour, and high on the glycemic index and therefore unhealthy for us. I wrote a whole book about carbohydrates, "The Good Carbohydrate Revolution" (Pocket Books 2002) and one of the most important messages of it was about the importance of the change in glycemic and insulin effects when food is ground up or processed into a powder or juice.

I believe that this concept is so important to the Peace Diet, I am repeating these graphs in case anyone may have missed them in the section on health and blood sugar control. In the chart below, you can see that when you turn rice into flour or potato into flour, it makes blood sugar increase even if you have the same amount of calories and grams of carbohydrate.

Blood Sugar Response to Different Forms of Carbohydrate

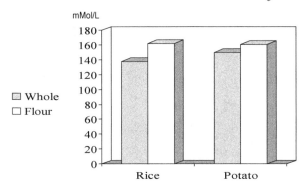

Crapo PA, Henry RR. *Am J Clin Nutr* 1988; 48:560 .

What is even worse, when you eat processed carbohydrates is that the insulin required goes up even more than the blood sugar indicates. In fact, the blood sugar would rise much higher if not for the heroic effort of the pancreas to keep the sugar down with insulin. And remember that chronically high insulin levels contribute to metabolic syndrome with weight gain, high blood pressure, and high triglycerides along with the high blood sugar.

Insulin Response to
Different Forms of Carbohydrate

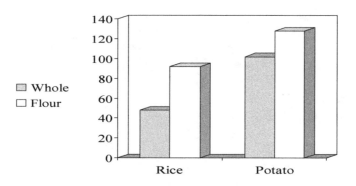

Crapo PA, Henry RR. A*m J Clin Nutr* 1988; 48:560 .

Some examples of whole grains include brown rice, steel cut oats, rolled oats, (never instant oats) buckwheat, quinoa, barley, corn, bulgur wheat, wild rice, millet, and rye. It is preferable to eat these grains cooked from whole or cracked kernels.

Processed grains should be used sparingly if at all, and they should be as minimally processed as possible. Also, pasta in general has a lower glycemic effect than does bread. For example, whole wheat pasta would be better than white pasta. Stone-ground bread whose flour particle size is much larger than that of commercially produced bread would be better than commercially produced whole wheat bread or white bread.

Paleolithic Diet: A Diet of Short Lifespan?

Some controversy exists about the use of grains as an optimal part of a healthy diet because humans lived in the Paleolithic era for over 100,000 years, and grains were introduced as a major part of the human diet only around 15,000 years ago. The thinking is that we are best adapted to a diet with little or no grains.

The problem with this reasoning is that Paleolithic humans lived only an estimated 25 to 35 years.[70]   I'm not saying such a diet causes early death. I'm saying that there is no way to use a Paleolithic diet as a model of eating for long life because they didn't live long enough to prove that it is compatible with long life. In addition, the human species never really thrived on earth in Paleolithic times. Only after introducing grains to our way of eating did humans begin to extend their life span and to thrive as a species on earth.

The Peace Diet is Healthy with or without Gluten for Most

Another issue that may be of concern is the gluten in some grains. Gluten is a grain protein that is found in wheat and related grains such as rye, barley and spelt. Some people are allergic to gluten and some have "celiac disease," a severe autoimmune reaction to gluten that may cause bleeding and damage to the digestive tract.

Another broader concern is that one of the components of gluten, called gliadin, can cause a disruption of the junctions between cells of the intestine and allow some large molecules to get through. This can result in an allergic, inflammatory, or autoimmune response to the invasion of these proteins into the blood stream. This is known popularly as "leaky gut syndrome." Some believe that this is a key to a number of health conditions such as allergies, autoimmune disease, arthritis, diabetes, and other inflammation-related diseases. In only a very small number of people is this verifiably a real problem and is real effect is due to the avoidance of processed carbohydrates. In addition, a gap in the gluten-free approach is that it usually ignores the fact that meat and saturated fat may also be causing inflammation due to "leaky gut,"[71]   and these foods are not reduced.

The best true estimates of the percentage of people with wheat allergy is approximately 0.1% or one out of a thousand. True celiac disease, a disease of autoimmunity due to gluten one out of effects about 0.7% of the population or about one out of 140 people. Non-celiac gluten sensitivity is estimated to be about 1% or one out of a hundred.[72]

Gluten May Not Be The Culprit

In a double-blind placebo-controlled study, gluten by itself had no effect on symptoms beyond placebo effect in participants when poorly digested short-chain carbohydrates were reduced. In other words, it appears that some of what is known as "gluten sensitivity" is placebo effect, and some of the symptoms may be caused by certain carbohydrates that are poorly absorbed which may change the gut flora.

Gluten vs Placebo Symptoms

After Reduction of Short-Chain Carbohydrates,
Gluten Has No Effect Beyond Placebo Effect

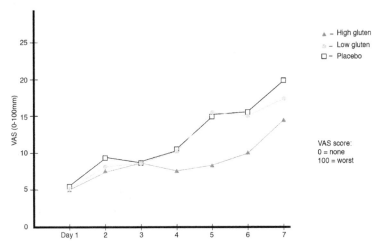

Adapted From: Biesiekierski JR, Peters SL, Newnham ED, et al. No effects of gluten in patients with self-reported non-celiac gluten sensitivity after dietary reduction of fermentable, poorly absorbed, short-chain carbohydrates. Gastroenterology 2013 145(2):320 - 8 - e1 – 3.

In my experience with the Peace Diet, I have seen allergies, asthma, autoimmune disease, arthritis, and diabetes resolve, whether or not gluten was included in the diet. In my programs, despite the fact that gluten-based meat substitutes, wheat berries, sprouted grain bread, stone-ground wheat tortillas, and barley are included, I still get participants off their diabetes medication, asthma medication, reduce joint pain, and resolve some autoimmune conditions such as psoriasis, and ulcerative colitis.

I believe that factors other than gluten, such as the avoidance of processed carbohydrates, account for the better control of blood sugar when wheat products are avoided.   Another factor to consider is the presence of the herbicide glyphosate (Roundup®). This herbicide is not just used as a weed killer. It is often sprayed directly on ripened wheat as a "dessicant" or "drying agent" to make it easier to harvest. Glyphosate is known to have a greater ability to disrupt tight junctions in the gut than gluten and can potentiate this effect. In addition, glyphosate is also patented as an antibiotic – not just as an herbicide. This means that it has the ability to disrupt your gut flora or your "microbiome". This is why I do use wheat products and gluten-containing products as long as they are "organic" (by definition herbicide-free).

Beans

The category of beans occupies the lower right-hand portion of the peace plate. It represents about 15 to 20% of the suggested intake and is a major source of the protein in the peace diet. Besides protein, beans provide a good balancing mix of macronutrients and fiber. For example, pinto beans are approximately 25% protein, 71% carbohydrate, and 4% fat. In addition, beans are an excellent source of fiber. For example, one cup of pinto beans provides approximately 10g of fiber. Some examples of foods in this category include pinto beans, kidney beans, black beans, garbanzo beans, (chickpeas), lentils, peas, lima beans, and soybeans.

Of all foods examined, the consumption of beans is the most important predictor of long life according to researchers.[73] Japanese eat soybeans, tofu, miso, black beans and azuki beans. The Swedes eat brown beans and peas, and in the Mediterranean diets, lentils, chickpeas (garbanzo beans), and white beans are commonly used. This association with long-life makes sense because beans are also known to have a number of health benefits such as cardiovascular protection.[74] There is also evidence that the consumption of beans can help control blood sugar and reduce the risk of diabetes II.[75]

Vegetarian Animals have Bigger Muscles Than Meat-Eaters
This has been true for more than 150,000,000 years

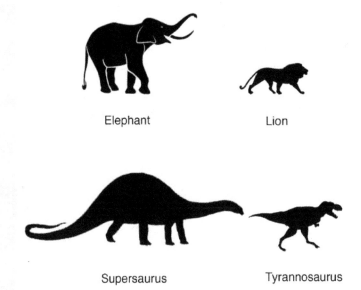

Elephant   Lion

Supersaurus   Tyrannosaurus

Protein

Beans and legumes provide an excellent source of protein. The truth is that grains are also a good source of protein, and so are vegetables. It is a misconception that plant-based proteins are somehow inferior to animal-based protein, and that a combining of plant-based sources of protein was necessary to provide an adequate amount of essential amino acids, which are the building blocks of protein. People say this all the time, and yet I have never seen anyone, professional or not, demonstrate the truth of this myth.

Review the following table and see if you can find any beans, grains, or vegetables that are inadequate in protein or any of the essential amino acids. Bear in mind that the RDA level of protein at 50 gm has about a 20% to 30% margin of safety built into it. In other words, the true minimum requirement for total protein is more likely around 35 to 40 grams of protein.

PROTEIN AND AMINO ACID TABLE								
Protein (in gm) and Essential Amino Acids (in mg) Available in 2,200 Calories of Food (RDA for Adult Female)								
	Protein	Trypto	Threo	Isoleu	Leucine	Lysine	Methio	Phenyl	Valine
RDA Female	50	250	450	650	950	800	425	475	650
Rice, Brown	51	714	2130	2465	4815	2222	1308	3009	3414
Corn	73	542	3072	3072	8312	3283	1596	3584	4427
Rice, White	47	590	1809	2173	4170	1821	1181	1688	3077
Potato	46	776	1810	2047	2995	3017	776	2279	2801
Turnip	86	982	2768	4018	3661	3923	1250	1964	3214
Kale	110	1829	6768	9023	10548	9023	1402	7682	8231
Broccoli	220	2608	8151	9782	11738	12716	3043	7608	11520
Beans, Kidney	129	1467	6846	8946	13583	11736	1576	8726	9584
Beef	132	1994	7798	8016	14098	14838	4568	6965	8673
Cheese, Cheddar	179	1193	5497	9593	14805	12878	4052	8147	10316

You can see plainly that none of the beans, grains, or vegetables are inadequate in protein except for white rice and potato which are both very close and fall within the margin of safety in protein that they provide. In addition, you will notice that even white rice and potato are more than adequate in all essential amino acids. I also hear so many people say that they need to eat meat to build muscle because, after all, meat is the muscle of an animal. Whenever I hear this comment, I ask the question: "Would you eat brain to get smarter? - or eat eyeballs to see better?"

It's funny how so many people believe this nonsense about muscle without thinking how illogical it would be to eat brain to get smarter. Of course, our bodies are much more complex than just eating a part of an animal to gain that characteristic in us. In fact, if you look at the animal kingdom, think about which animals have the biggest muscles -- meat eaters or plant eaters. In nature, plant-eaters such as elephants have much bigger muscles than meat eaters such as lions. In fact, this has been true for at least 150 million years since the time of the "brontosaurus" (now called Apatosaurus or or Supersaurus).   While protein is an important contribution of beans to a healthy diet, you might notice that the main component of beans is carbohydrate. Beans are a wonderfully low-glycemic source of carbohydrates to go along with the carbohydrates you can get from grains. For example, the glycemic index number for beans are typically somewhere between 30 and 50.

Beans	100 grams				calories %		
	calories	fat	carbs	protein	fat	carbs	protein
Pinto	143	0.7	26	9	4%	72%	24%
Black	132	0.5	24	9	3%	72%	26%
Soy (edamame)	122	5	10	11	35%	30%	35%
Garbanzo	164	2.6	27	9	14%	65%	21%
Lentils	116	0.4	20	9	3%	67%	30%
Lima	115	0.4	21	8	3%	71%	26%
Navy	140	0.6	26	8	4%	74%	22%
Kidney	127	0.5	23	9	3%	70%	27%

*fat, carbs, and protein in grams.

Nuts

Nuts are also part of the "Beans" group because they are high in protein, and some beans or legumes cross over into the "Nut" family.   A good example is peanuts. The difference is that nuts are much higher in fat than beans. See the table below:

	100 grams				calories %		
	calories	fat	carbs	protein	fat	carbs	protein
Chestnuts	213	2	46	2	9%	87%	4%
Cashews	553	44	33	18	69%	20%	11%
Pistachio	557	44	28	21	70%	18%	12%
Peanuts	567	49	16	26	75%	9%	16%
Almonds	575	49	22	21	74%	14%	12%
Hazelnuts	628	61	17	15	84%	9%	7%
Walnuts	654	65	14	15	85%	7%	8%
Brazil nuts	656	66	12	14	87%	6%	7%
Pine nuts	673	68	13	14	87%	6%	7%
Pecans	691	72	14	9	91%	6%	3%
Macadamia	718	76	14	8	93%	5%	3%

*fat, carbs, and protein in grams.

Vitamin B-12

B12 is the one nutrient that you can't really get efficiently from plants. It is essential for the production of blood, it supports the nervous system, and the body needs it. But you need very little of it, and most people who are vegetarian still will eat some foods that have B12 in them, when they are not strict vegetarians.

Part of the B-12 deficiency may occur in both vegans and meat-eaters because that our food may be too clean. Of course, we have to wash our food these days because of possible contaminations in the soil. However, in ancient times, we did eat some dirt that came along with vegetables and roots that allowed us to obtain B-12 from the bacteria that lives symbiotically with root systems. This is how some herbivores obtain their B-12 in a natural way. From good soil, we can also obtain other useful nutrients that are not found in foods such as humic and fulvic acid. B-12 is also found in mushrooms and in trace amounts in fermented foods and some seaweeds.

Nevertheless, if you are a strict vegan, you should periodically check the B12 level in your bloodstream. If you wish to take a vitamin B12 supplement as a caution against deficiency, they are simple to get, and you can also get B-12 in some fortified cereals.

Fruit

On the left side of the peace plate, the lower portion consists of fruit and is roughly 15 to 20% of the plate. Fruit is a category that is usually the easiest to fulfill for most people because it is usually eaten as a single food and often in its raw unprocessed form. For example apples, oranges, pears, and cherries are usually eaten raw. For the purpose of the peace plate, fresh whole fruit whether raw or cooked is the preferred food for this category. You have to be careful if you are considering canned fruit because most of it is packed in sugar-laden syrup.

Fruit is important on the peace diet because, like vegetables, it is loaded with powerful vitamins and micronutrients. Fruits are also a good source of fiber and are high on my mass index scale, so they help make you feel full and naturally limit your calorie intake. Some of the beneficial nutrients found in fruit are as follows:

Apples:
triterpenoids and quercetin (in the skin of the apple) - a group of anticancer nutrients
Blueberries, Blackberries, Cherries, Acai Berries: Anthocyanins - powerful antioxidants
Guavas, Oranges, Strawberries:
vitamin C, bioflavonoids - anti-cancer properties
Grapes, Blueberries:
resveratrol – known to have a cardio-protective effect
Pomegranate:
punicaligin - anti-atherosclerotic
Peaches, Apricots, Cantaloupe:

beta-carotene - antioxidant associated with lower risk of certain cancers

Mangoes:

Lutein, zeaxanthin - antioxidants associated with prevention of macular degeneration and heart disease

There is a caution about fruit. The fruit section is smaller than the vegetable or grain section because it is possible to get too much sugar from eating large quantities of fruit. This is especially a problem with tropical fruit such as bananas and figs because their glycemic index is relatively high. Juicing fruit will increase the glycemic index of the fruit and worsen its impact on blood sugar. Also, be aware that the sugar in fruit is mainly fructose. Fructose has less of an effect on blood sugar than glucose or table sugar, which is half glucose and half fructose; however, it is worse for triglycerides and LDL, the bad cholesterol.

Beverages

Beverages should be water or non-caloric beverages such as tea or herbal tea. Be sure to avoid sugared drinks and even more so, artificially sweetened drinks. Ironically, sugar-free is worse than sugar because they add chemicals such as aspartame, sucralose and saccharin to sweeten "sugar free" beverages. If you are going to try any sugar substitute, use stevia because it is a natural glycoside from the *stevia rebaudiana* plant originally from Paraguay.

Fruit should be eaten whole. Pure fruit juices are, of course, better than sugared or artificially sweetened beverages but the problem is, as you turn fruit into juice, you raise the glycemic index number of the fruit.

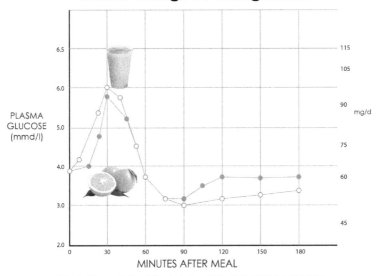

Blood Sugar Response to Whole Orange vs Orange Juice

Adapted from: Bolton RP, et al, Am J Clin Nutr 1981;34:211-217

For example, in comparing oranges and orange juice, the blood sugar response to orange juice (white dots) is slightly higher than that of oranges. But later you see that there is a slow return to normal blood sugar. This is bordering on hypoglycemia or low blood sugar later. This low sugar can lead to fatigue, hunger and cravings.

What's worse is that juicing fruit makes the insulin go even higher. As I explained earlier in this book, high insulin levels contribute to metabolic syndrome. In the following graph, it is clear that drinking orange juice causes insulin to go much higher than eating whole oranges.

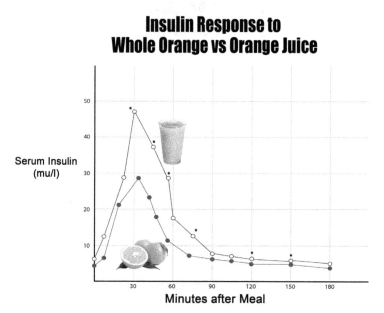

Insulin Response to
Whole Orange vs Orange Juice

Serum Insulin (mu/l)

Minutes after Meal

Adapted from: Bolton RP, et al, Am J Clin Nutr 1981;34:211-217

If you want to do juicing, add lots of vegetables to reduce the glycemic number of the juice. And remember that carrots, although very healthy and full of carotenoids and excellent nutrition, have a glycemic number higher than plain sugar and, though eating them is usually not a problem because they are just seven grams of carbs per carrot, juicing carrots could easily give you too much sugar.

If you are going to drink caffeinated beverages, tea is preferable to coffee because tea is alkalizing and also has some known anti-cancer and anti-inflammatory processes. Coffee is okay for health, but it can be acidifying. Further, it can contribute to afternoon tiredness and needs to be excluded in the regimen of spiritual development. What is even better is tea that does not have caffeine in it. Most herbal teas are very good for this purpose. Hawaiian mamaki tea is known to have similar anti-cancer phytonutrients as green tea but has no caffeine in it.

Summary

In summary, I take the round plate, split it down the middle and draw a peace sign. The upper left section or 30 to 35% of the plate would be for vegetables, emphasizing dark leafy greens and sea vegetables for calcium, and a variety of colorful yellow, orange and red vegetables for antioxidants and pigments. The lower left section of the "Peace Plate" or about 15% to 20% of the plate is for fruit in a smaller amount than vegetables. Then on the right half of the plate, about 60%, 70% on the right hand side (or 30 to 35% of the whole plate) would be whole grain with little if any highly processed grains. And at the bottom the rest of the plate would be beans and legumes for a good source of protein, fiber and low-glycemic carbohydrate. To not mislead people, it is not called "protein," as in the USDA "My Plate" because protein is found in all 4 groups of food.

Dr. Shintani's
Whole Person
Peace Plan

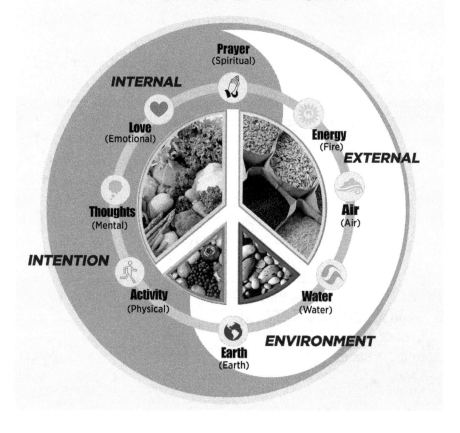

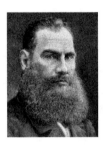

*"If a man earnestly seeks a
righteous life, his first act of
abstinence is from animal food..."
-LEO TOLSTOY (1828-1910)*

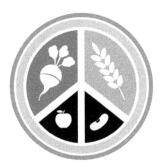

VI- THE WHOLE PERSON PEACE DIET PLAN

As organisms, our well-being does not depend on working as little as possible, but on activating all our forces. Rudolf Steiner[76]

The Peace Diet is not just a diet of food. It is about all that we take in. This includes food, herbs, chemicals, water, air, energy, thoughts and spiritual energy.

In Chapter II, the fifth main lesson is that it is not just about food. There are environmental factors that affect health, and there are also internal factors that also have an effect on health. I have divided them into 8 factors that I display around the plate. Part of the reason for this is that I believe that diet is the most important factor, so the plate is at the center of the diagram. I have further categorized them into four external factors and four internal factors.

The external factors are represented by earth, air, energy and water. These correspond to the ancient four elements of alchemy.

We need to be sure that we are exposed to the right kind and amount of solid substances (food, herbs, supplements, chemicals), clean air, energy (eg, sunlight, radiation), and clean water. The four internal factors are based on our own intentions. They are exercise, thoughts, love and prayer. These correspond to the four elements of whole person health; physical, mental, emotional and spiritual health practices. While I believe that diet is the most important determinant of your health, these eight other aspects are also important contributors to your overall health.

Dr. Shintani's
Whole Person
Peace Plan

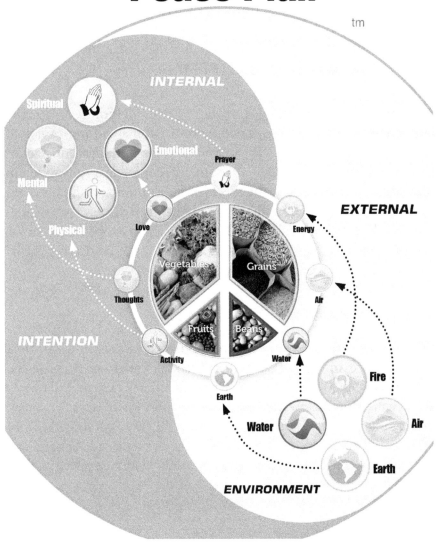

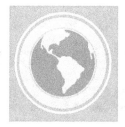

Earth

The first environmental exposure we will describe is "Earth" because we are covering our exposure to atoms and molecules of all kinds that are in their solid phase. This includes substances that are large and smaller than microscopic. For example, in descending order of size, the kinds of substances to which we are exposed include food, herbs, supplements, hormones, natural and unnatural molecules, and minerals. As with all exposures, there is the optimal type, quantity and proportion and even the best of substances can be harmful if taken in excess.

Food

Of course, we have already been describing in detail our greatest connection to the earth , which is through our food because the food becomes us. We are literally what we eat. Our whole body is virtually completely replaced over a period of up to 7 years, depending on what tissue is involved. And although most but not all cells are replaced, the atoms in them are replaced. Therefore, we truly are what we eat. So, our physical health depends mainly on what we consume.

Based on a report by the American Academy of Environmental Medicine (AAEM), another serious threat to our health may be GMO food. Based on their scientific analysis, there should be a moratorium on GMO food until long term testing for safety is done.[74]   Most of the countries in the world agree that safety studies need to be done. However, the chemical companies who benefit have created political and PR campaigns to suggest their GMO products are safe. But there are no long-term studies to show that they are safe, and there is ample evidence that GMO food has caused harm to animals and insects according to the AAEM.

Proponents obscure this concern by claiming that there is no "science" that GMO products cause harm to humans. However, what people should be asking is 'where is the science that it is safe in the long run?'. There is clear evidence that the GMO process of producing L-Tryptophan in the 1990's likely caused deaths through "eosinophilia myalgia syndrome."[78]   Essentially, we are in the same place we were in the early days of the tobacco industry where they claimed that smoking was not harmful. We now have millions of deaths to prove that it is, and for the deceased, it is too late. We should learn from this horrible experience. If the canary has died in the mineshaft, should we go in just because we have no proof that humans will die? Where are the science and the proof that in the long run, GMO foods are safe?

We also want to not over-consume certain foods such as foods that may cause allergies. For example, there is some concern that gluten is a problem for many people. However, this has probably been over-emphasized and in reality, relatively few people actually have problems with gluten and the problems solved by avoiding gluten are largely the result of avoiding processed wheat flour. In contrast, many more people have problems likely caused by too many animal products and dairy; these include heart disease, stroke and certain cancers. Ironically, many people avoid gluten and consume more meat without realizing that meat intake can also cause leaky gut syndrome.[79]

Soy is another example of a food of possible concern - even if it is non-GMO. Research on the Okinawans showed that their long life-span was related to their un-processed food diet which included about 2 to 4 oz. of soy, usually in the form of tofu and miso every day. This amount should be fine for most people; however, consuming much more than that may allow it to have an anti-thyroid effect by blocking an enzyme that allows for the production of thyroid hormone. There are other vegetables that can do that when eaten in large quantities, especially when uncooked.

Herbs

Besides food, we are also consuming the earth in other ways, for example, through herbs. As we all know, many of the foods we eat are also herbs and in some ways, all herbs are also foods. Some simple examples are garlic, ginger, turmeric, green tea, and Hawaiian mamaki tea. I also mention the use of herbal teas in the "Water" section of the eight enhancements to the diet for whole person health. We can optimize our health by using healing herbs but, of course, that is a subject worthy of another book. I consider herbs to be different from supplements because herbs are whole plants, and supplements are molecules separated from plants.

Supplements

Another entire book could be written about supplements as well. When we think of supplements, the most common of them are vitamins. Vitamins are those substances other than basic calories and water that our bodies cannot do without. For example, the lack of vitamin C led to scurvy among British sailors. The lack of vitamin B1 (thiamin) led to beriberi among Japanese sailors. Supplements are generally substances extracted from plants that are useful or even necessary for health such as vitamins and other substances that may not be considered vitamins. A common example of this is Co-enzyme Q-10 which is not a vitamin because your body makes plenty of it, but is useful to the body in energy production and may be useful in congestive heart failure.

Nutrition from the Earth

While our greatest intake from the Earth is through food that we eat, we also can obtain nutrition from directly consuming tiny amounts of earth directly. The most obvious nutrition that we get directly or indirectly from the Earth is in the form of minerals. Minerals are atomic elements and therefore cannot be manufactured by plants, although plants absorb minerals and we get most of our minerals through plants. We should be sure that our intake of minerals is appropriate; this includes the right amounts of calcium, iron, iodine, selenium, magnesium, chromium and so forth.

There are also substances besides minerals that are in the Earth that may be important for our nutrition. In India there is a legend that near the Himalaya mountains, when the weather became warmer during the approach of summer, monkeys would go into the mountains and come down energized and strong. When curious observers followed some of the monkeys, they found them licking a black tarry substance that was oozing out of the rocks in the mountainside.

For thousands of years, this subsance known as "shilajit" has been used for numerous ailments in Ayurvedic medicine, including restoration of energy and as an antiseptic. There is some early research on its use for restoration of cognitive function.[80]   The active substances in Shilagit appear to be humic acid and fulvic acid. These are substances that are the by-product of the degradation of plants and micro-organisms. They appear to assist in the absorption of other nutrients into the cells and thereby improve cellular function.

Vitamin B-12 is another nutrient that may be found in the soil. It is the only vitamin not produced by plant or animal. Earlier in this book we discussed how vitamin B-12 is found generally in animal products and mushrooms. In the soil it is found near the roots of plants. It is formed by soil bacteria in a symbiotic relationship to the plants. It is also found in soil that is fertilized by manure and compost. In ancient times, B-12 was likely obtained through the consumption of root vegetables or mushrooms. Today, we are perhaps too fastidiously clean with our vegetables and probably don't eat enough mushrooms, so we may need B-12 supplementation if a vegan diet is followed strictly and animal products are completely avoided.

Drugs and Chemicals

It is important to remember that while medications are useful, too much of a good thing or the wrong combination of things can be dangerous. I put drugs and chemicals in the same category because they are generally not natural to the human body and in general do not bring people to good health. What is of great concern is the fact that medications - even properly prescribed - have been reported to be the fourth leading cause of death in the U.S. as a result of adverse reactions to them.

Of course, medications are necessary in many cases to prevent the damage from diseases such as high blood pressure and diabetes. However, the simple fact that people have to remain on these medications should tell you that medications never create optimal health and by definition, a person who relies on medication is still sick in some way. For good health, it is important to look for the cause of the disease and deal with that before putting people on a lot of chronic medication.

Toxic Chemicals

Obviously, it is important to avoid the intake of toxins and outright poisons such as herbicides, pesticides, cleaning chemicals, radioactive materials, and so forth. We also want to limit our intake of harmful elements such as mercury, lead, arsenic, hexavalent chromium (as in the movie "Erin Brockovitch"), cadmium and berylium. We need to also limit exposure to substances that may seem helpful at times such as fluoride and chlorine, both of which can block normal thyroid function by replacing iodine in thyroid hormone production. This may render the hormone inactive and result in fatigue and hypothyroid symptoms in the face of normal thyroid.

There are many man-made chemicals in our environment that have been used in our soils and fields for agriculture and industry; they have been accumulating over many years. The problems caused by such chemicals also known as "Persistent Organic Pollutants" or POPs are numerous; they include cancers, birth defects, hormone changes, and probably a slew of unknown diseases. Remember that such toxic environmental pollutants will be bio-concentrated in animal products. This is another way that the Peace Diet contributes to your health by limiting animal products. No matter what you might hear about pollution of food and the water supply, remember that pollution is amplified in animal products because many of the toxins get stored up and accumulated in animal fat. For more detail, read the book "What the Health" by Dr. D. Nomura, soon to be available at lulu.com.

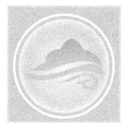

Air

For breath is life, and if you breathe well you will live long on earth.
~Sanskrit Proverb

Our second area of environmental exposure is air, which we need to breathe. We take the importance of clean air for granted as it is readily available from our first breath as an infant to our last breath on the day we leave this Earth.

We take it for granted unless we are exposed to polluted air. I can't tell you how many patients I have whose allergies act up when there is smog in the air. They report problems like shortness of breath, asthma, fatigue, sinus congestion and more. In Hawaii, we are also faced with vog - or volcanic fog which comes from the active volcanoes on the big island of Hawaii.

Breathe Clean Air

The absolute worst insult to the quality of the air we breathe is smoking. It is a testament to the importance of clean air. Millions of deaths are attributable to smoking. Smoking not only contributes to lung disease and cancer, it is a major contributor to heart disease by causing inflammation and scarring in the arteries thereby accelerating coronary heart disease and strokes. Only recently have we begun to realize how bad secondhand smoke is for people's health. There is now a lot of evidence that secondhand smoke is associated with higher risks of heart disease, allergies, and several forms of cancer. Of course, the primary smoker is at much higher risk for these diseases.

Airborne pollutants can also come from cars, machinery and industry. The air can carry aerosolized toxic chemicals for miles and miles. One of the most egregious examples of this was the use of Agent Orange as a defoliant in Vietnam during the Vietnam war. Only years later was it seen that this was the likely cause of horrific birth defects in Vietnamese babies and diseases among our own soldiers. It is possible that such accidents are happening even now in Hawaii where they are testing powerful pesticides in fields near public schools. What is of great concern is that there is no science based on long-term testing that shows this to be a safe practice.

Breathing for Optimal Health

Breathing air properly, as simple and mundane as it may sound, may be the simplest and yet most important neglected thing we can do.   Think about the word "spirit." It is derived from the Latin word "spiritus" or "breath" in English.   This being the case, how could breathing not be important to the health of the spirit? In the ancient Hawaiian tradition, the word "ha" means "breath of life," which refers to the essence of life that resides in one's body.   One of the first lessons taught by practitioners of traditional Hawaiian healing is proper breathing.

In the tradition of the Shaolin monks, breathing was considered essential in all aspects of their training. One description of the importance of breathing comes from the "Wisdom of the Temple of Zen."

> *At the Shaolin Temple, the monks know how important the breath is. Every movement they do, every kick, every punch is done with the breath of Qi. They are famous throughout the world for increasing their martial power and the rate of their health and longevity through a series of breathing exercise called Qigong.*[81]

Grand-Master Dr. Effie Chow, former presidential advisor to the National Institutes of Health for the National Center for Complementary and Alternative Medicine and founder of East West Academy of Healing Arts, always teaches the importance of breathing in her Qigong classes.   She points out that the most fundamental currency that supports the Qi, the life-force is breathing.   She says: *"After all, without breath there is no life."*

This is also true in Ayurvedic healing practices as well. In meditation, it is always important to sit straight up with your back straight and with your feet flat on the ground. Sitting straight is important because it allows the "bellows" action of your lungs in breathing air in and out to be maximized. This helps you to meditate and to start your day because breathing properly alkalizes the blood. Alkalizing your blood will help to boost the cellular voltage in your body. This will help your entire body function at a higher level. It will also enhance your meditation by giving your brain enough oxygen and energy to make use of its full potential.

> *When we breathe—breathe in, breathe out—we create a connection between our inner source and its outward manifestation.*
> Kealapono, Teacher of Meditation

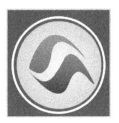

Water

The third important environmental exposure is water. As with air and food, we can't live without water. We are 70% water by weight and water is vital to circulation and all our cellular functions. When you think about it, life itself started in the oceans even without air. On Earth, life (not human or animal life) is possible without air but not without water; so, clean water is the basic medium of physical life.

Clean water is currently an important issue. More and more drinking water is being contaminated by environmental pollutants of all kinds; for example, pesticides and herbicides that are used on farms eventually find their way down into the water table and, to some extent, are made worse by the use of GMO (Genetically Modified Organism) crops. These crops are herbicide-resistant and therefore require the use of more and more herbicide to control weeds because the crops tolerate higher amounts. Eventually, herbicides as well as pesticides leach into groundwater and contaminate drinking water and water used on food crops. After all, these chemicals have to go somewhere.

Fluoridation and chlorination of water is another important concern in relation to clean drinking water. One of the unforeseen problems with fluoridation is the effect on thyroid hormones. Because fluoride is a halogen like iodine, it can replace iodine in the production of thyroid hormone. This would render the thyroid hormone inactive and reduce the amount of active thyroid in the blood stream. This could cause symptoms of low thyroid such as fatigue, mild depression, and weight gain, even though blood levels of thyroid are normal.

Beverages

Another important issue in relation to water intake is our consumption of beverages instead of plain water. One of the biggest culprits for the high rate of diabetes and obesity in the US is the over-consumption of sugar-laden soft drinks. What's worse is that the most popular solution to this problem is the use of artificial sweeteners such as aspartame (such as NutraSweet ®) and sucralose (such as Splenda ®). Studies have shown potential side effects such as weight gain and cancer. Further, no long-term studies have shown that either sweetener is completely safe. As for fruit juices and milk, most people don't realize that calories in the form of beverages tend to hit the bloodstream much faster than calories from food. This can contribute to diabetes and obesity. For this reason, calorie-containing beverages are to be limited and water and tea are preferred.

In fact, getting water in the form of tea can be very healing. There are a number of teas that are like herbal medicine or at least have some health value. For example, simple green tea has been shown to have significant anti-cancer nutrients in them such as polyphenols, catechins, and flavonoids. Oolong tea (which is camellia sinensis, the same species as green and black tea) has been demonstrated to help increase metabolism and induce a small amount of weight loss. All the green teas have caffeine in them. Hawaii also has a unique tea called Mamaki that has all the same anti-cancer nutrients as green tea -- the polyphenols, catechins and flavonoids but without any caffeine.

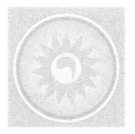

Energy

The most pervasive environmental exposure is energy, to which we are exposed 24/7. It comes from the sun, the universe and elements all around us. The heat and radiation from the sun exposes us to electromagnetic radiation including light and frequencies beyond visible light. We are also exposed to electromagnetic fields from the Earth as well (the earth's electromagnetic pulsing frequency is 7.8 cycles per second). We are also exposed to cosmic energy from the stars and radiation from the stars and from the earth.

We need the right exposure to energy of all kinds. For example, when we optimize our exposure to sunlight, we get vitamin D. There is also evidence that the pulsing of the Earth's magnetic field is necessary for optimal health. If we are exposed to the wrong energy, like radiation, we will get DNA damage, which could result in cancer or other health problems. If we are exposed to too much heat or sunlight, we get sunburn or possibly worse.

Some of the newer threats to our health in regard to energy exposure come about because of our modernizing society. Radiation from nuclear reactors and accidents at these types of facilities such as Chernobyl and the Fukushima Daiichi disaster is just one example. Another new threat is also cell phone energy that we put right up to our ears. For a more in-depth explanation of this subject, read the book, "What the Health" by Dr. D Nomua, co-host of my radio show. The book may be available soon at www.lulu.com, and the radio show may be heard on the website www.kwai1080hi.com on Sunday nights at 8 pm Hawaii Time.

Healing Energy

Energy is also a healing medium. When we have health issues such as wounds, aches and pains, or injured muscles, we may need some help in optimizing healing. The concept of energy medicine was pioneered in the earliest days of the Ayurvedic and Traditional Chinese Medicine traditions. The belief is that there is energy flowing through the body through meridians, and illness and pain are due to an imbalance in the energy. Acupuncture achieves its results by stimulating or dampening this energy, whichever is appropriate through the use of acupuncture points on the skin. Acupressure is based on the same principles. Other "energy healing techniques such as Reiki and Okada Purifying Therapy, which includes delivering healing energy through a technique known as Jorei, and Traditional Hawaiian Healing techniques have been demonstrated to be surprisingly useful.

Healing and Voltage

In general agreement with this ancient concept, Dr. Jerry Tennant, a distinguished ophthalmologist and energy medicine pioneer wrote a book called, "Healing Is Voltage." In this book, he describes the concept that aches, pains and dysfunction in our bodies could be healed if we had enough voltage in our cells to repair and produce new cells. He developed a device known as the "Tennant Biomodulator" that appears to be very useful in helping to reduce pain and improve a number of conditions in the body.

There are now numerous energy modalities that are effective as therapy for a number of conditions. There has long been the use of "pulsed electro-magnetic fields" (PEMF) and "transcutaneous electrical nerve stimulation" (TENS) units for chronic pain and other conditions. On the cutting edge currently are technologies such as low level lasers as well as "light emitting diode" (LED) therapies.

Scalar Energy

Scalar energy is a type of energy that was predicted to exist by James Clerk Maxwell, one of the discoverers of electro-magnetic fields, and Nikola Tesla, the inventor of alternating current. It is a type of energy field that doesn't point in any direction - unlike electro-magnetic fields which has a definite directionality. Vector fields such as gravity and electro-magnetic fields have both magnitude and direction. Scalar fields just have magnitude just as temperature has magnitude but no directionality. The importance of this difference becomes apparent when we look at the effect of electromagnetic fields (EMF) and the potentially harmful effects of electromagnetic equipment such as computers, radios, stereos, cell phones, and transformers. Scalar energy fields appear to have the potential of cancelling such negative fields and imparting energy into living cells.

Of some special interest are scalar energy field generators such as the EES or Energy Enhancement System developed by Dr. Sandra Rose Michael. This concept may be an important part of the future of medicine.

People should be skeptical, however, because many systems claim to be "scalar" but few can document their production. Some of the effects of optimizing bodily energy through scalar fields are quite remarkable. We have published a peer-reviewed case study on the mitigation of seizures using this energy system.[82] Uniquely, this energy system has been confirmed to be creating scalar energy fields by Dr. John Orava, a high-level Department of Defense biophysics consultant.

This rounds out our environmental exposures to what might be compared to the ancient alchemy elements Earth, Air, Fire (energy), and Water. The next four items or factors that can enhance our health are based on our own intention. They are Activity, Thoughts, Love, and Prayer, which also correspond to the physical, mental, emotional and spiritual aspects of your being.

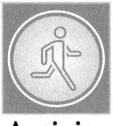

Activity

Exercise

"An early-morning walk is a blessing for the whole day"

Henry David Thoreau

The next important aspect of our health is activity. We need to exercise to optimize our health and to give us the best chance of avoiding disease and mental decline. Next to diet, physical activity is the most important thing you can do to maintain the health of your body and mind. Study after study indicates that people who exercise regularly have lower rates of heart disease, diabetes, cancer, Alzheimer's disease, and premature death.

My radio show co-host Dr. Ruth Heidrich was featured on the documentary "Forks Over Knives.. She is a great example of a person reversing aging and disease. She is a long-term survivor of breast cancer. She is vegan, consuming no dairy and her bone density goes up every year. She gets up every morning and takes an early morning run and bikes and swims nearly every day. You would never guess that she is nearly 80 years old.

Lose Weight While You Sleep

Want to lose weight while you sleep? You can if you take a few simple actions daily to get some regular exercise. There are some simple things you can do to help control your weight and improve your health, and they are not about dieting. One of the best ways to be active is to choose something physically active to do that is fun. After all, when, exactly, did exercise become work? Think about it. As a child you ran and played, and your fat furnace was in overdrive to burn enough energy to keep up with you. You kept your muscles in tone, kept your cardiovascular system fit, burned calories like a well-oiled machine, and enjoyed every moment of it! And there's no reason why you can't learn again right now to enjoy exercising. There are three main kinds of exercise that we should include for optimal health. They are what I call the "three S's." That would be Stamina, Strength and Stretching.

Exercise for Stamina

Regular aerobic activity (the kind that makes you breathe faster and your heart rate go up) is one step to helping you "lose weight while you sleep." These kinds of activity help you build stamina. Aerobic activities include many of the things you may already love to do like running, skiing, swimming, and a thousand other things you can surely think of. Aerobic exercise allows you to burn calories as well as burn fat! (10) Start with at least 30 minutes every other day. Try to move up to at least 40 minutes every other day.

If you can exercise in this way an average of four times per week for 30 to 40 minutes, directly burning calories isn't the only benefit of exercising. In fact, now, the main effect of exercising takes place when we are not exercising at all! Let's say that you exercise three to four times per week. This causes your metabolism to increase at all times. This, in turn, means that your Resting Metabolic Rate - the rate at which you burn calories while you're at rest - and even sleep - increases at all times, as a result of the regular exercise. This means it helps you to lose weight while you sleep.

Strength Exercise

Strength exercise is also important in helping you to keep your ideal body weight. Muscle cells, even if they are inactive, burn an average of 13 calories per kilogram per day while fat cells burn an average of only 4.5 calories per kilogram per day (8). When muscle cells become active they, of course, burn even more than they do at rest.

In other words, muscles burn about three times as many calories as fat does when they are at rest and when you are asleep. Thus, it stands to reason that the more muscle mass you have on your body and the less fat mass, the more calories you will burn at all times, even in your sleep. So if you want to *help* your body burn energy and metabolize stored fat, you need to incorporate resistance-training activities that tone your body and build or at least retain muscle mass.

Get Comfortable With Strength Training

You'll notice in the paragraph above that I talk about your need to find 'activities' to tone your body. It isn't necessary to become a health club nut. If it's not practical for you, you don't have to get your workout at a gym…although a full cycle workout of your major muscle groups would not hurt.

If nothing else, do simple, home-based exercises that require strength, such as push-ups, sit-ups, or stair-stepping for starters.

Make strength training a part of your life, and you can retain the muscle mass that will help you burn calories faster and help you lose weight while you sleep.

Stretching Exercise

The third type of exercise that is important is quite simple. It is stretching. This simply means that once a day, you should move all your joints to their full range of motion. This helps to prevent injury and allows for full circulation of blood to areas and muscles that you don't ordinarily move much. It helps to prevent stagnation and makes sure that you don't lose any range of motion that might be limited because of not using your body to its fullest.

Some of the more formal exercise styles that do well with this include yoga, Pilates, and tai chi. If you don't have the time or inclination to do these types of exercises, you can do some simple home exercises. In martial arts classes, we used to do simple stretching from head to toe in the following order:

1. Rotate head from side to side - then roll it around tilting in all angles.
2. Rotate shoulders over and over in a shrugging motion. Then with your right hand, grab your left elbow and pull it towards your right shoulder. Then do the same with your left hand and pull the right elbow to the left shoulder.
3. Rotate arms in a windmill motion. End by interlocking fingers and raising your hands together palms up as high as you can go. Some people will "crack" their knuckles in this position.
4. Rotate at waist side to side.

5. Bend forward and touch your toes. Then bend back as far as you can and then bend forward again to touch your toes.
6. Put your hands on your knees and bend your knees together. Then move your knees and hands together in a clockwise motion. Then rotate in a clockwise motion.
7. Then step to the side with your right leg, bend your knee and turn your head and shoulders to the left. Squat down on your right leg and keeping your left heel in the ground, stretch the back of your left leg. Then do the same on the right.

Doing these exercises daily can help you to remain healthy and strong in all your joints and helps to prevent injury and loss of your ability to walk, sit, stand and perform other basic activities.

Sleep

In addition, we need to balance our activity with an appropriate amount of rest and sleep. As much as our bodies need exercise to maintain muscle and health, our bodies need rest to repair and to rejuvenate. For many people, sleep is an afterthought. The reality is that sleep can have a profound effect on our health in areas such as mental performance, depression, blood sugar control and weight control. Lack of sleep has been tied to increases in the hormone cortisol which can lead to and increase in weight. In addition, lack of sleep has been associated with an increase in ghrelin - a substance known to increase appetite.

Sleep also influences our immune system through the production of a hormone called melatonin. Melatonin is produced by the pineal gland which sits behind and above the pituitary gland and near the center of the brain. It is sometimes called the "third eye." As mystical as this may sound, in reality, the pineal gland, though not exposed to the surface, is extremely sensitive to light. It is said that the pineal gland connects us to the rhythms of the day and of the universe. Melatonin is optimized with regular sleep and when a person is exposed to light, somehow, the signal gets to the pineal gland and melatonin production is shut down.

Melatonin is probably best known as a sleep aid and can be taken as a supplement for sleep. More recently, there has been research that suggests that it may be important in the prevention of cancer. Blind women who could not perceive light were found to have 50% less breast cancer than those who could perceive light suggesting that they were protected due to optimized melatonin because light could not shut its production down. Melatonin is known to have potent anti-oxidative effects and can enhance the production of "natural killer cells" important in fighting cancer. In a meta-analysis of the use of melatonin in the treatment of cancer, researchers found a reduction in risk of death of 34% in one year. [83]

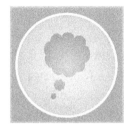

Thoughts

We are what we think. All that we are arises out of our thoughts. With our thoughts we make the world. . . . As the wheel follows the ox that draws the cart.

Ancient Buddhist Saying

To some extent, we are indeed a product of our own thoughts. There is evidence that our thoughts can have a profound effect on our physical health. There is a discipline in the field of medicine known as "psychoneuroimmunology," which studies and makes use of the connection between our mind and our ability to influence our health through our immune system. Intuitively, I think we all are aware that stress can affect our health. But psychoneuroimmunology is the study of how the mind (psycho) through our nervous system (neuro) can influence our ability to fight disease (immunology).

This field of study, also described as "Mind-Body Medicine," is now recognized as legitimate, and there are centers around the country devoted to this approach to healing such as the UCLA Cousins Center for Psychoneuroimmunology, and The Benson-Henry Institute for Mind-Body Medicine at Harvard University and many others.

Our thoughts can make a major impact on our health in other ways. Stress can cause hormonal changes such as a chronic elevation of a steroid hormone, cortisol. This can contribute to obesity and heart disease. Meditation is known to help lower their stress levels and reduce the risk of coronary heart disease and stroke. This is well documented in the literature, especially with mindful meditation and transcendental meditation.[84]

I have always believed in the saying by Ralph Waldo Emerson about the connection between our thoughts and our destiny. He once wrote:

> *Sow a thought, reap and action*
> *Sow an action, reap a habit*
> *Sow a habit, reap a character*
> *Sow a character, reap a destiny.*
> -Ralph Waldo Emerson

I believe this also applies to our health in terms of our health-related habits such as exercise, smoking, drinking, eating, sleeping, and thinking. All of this begins with our thoughts.

Our thoughts are also reflected in our words. Words have power. The Bible says that *"In the beginning there was the word and the word was with God and the word was God."* John 1:1

Of course, this refers to the word of God, but it also suggests that words have power. It is because words cause your mind to focus on a thought. Indeed, you are what you say as well as what you think. So, it is important to speak well of others.

Choose words very carefully. Words can be hurtful or can be inspiring. It helps our own health when we choose words wisely and speak well of others. It not only keeps our own minds positive, it also helps to improve our relationships and reduce stress in our lives.

The Rotary Club has a four way test of things that we think and do:

1. Is it is true?
2. It is fair to all concerned?
3. Is it beneficial to those involved?
4.   Will it help to build good relationships?

I think it is very wise to consider all four before you say things. In addition to fostering good relationships, it ends up relieving stress in the long run.

Subconscious Habit Change

Part of the reason it is so important to make the best use of our mind and our thoughts is because our thoughts create pictures in our minds. When we see pictures in our minds over and over, they make a take on our subconscious mind. This is where our habits are developed - in our subconscious mind. What is in our subconscious mind not only affects our immune system through the mind-body connection, it also affects our lifestyle habits of eating, drinking, exercise and so forth. This is how to make long term lifestyle changes stick and become the healthy habits that can change your health destiny.

Reaching the subconscious mind is used in self-hypnosis. Our subconscious mind is like our autopilot system. It is affected over time with repetition and with sensory and emotional cues. It is like a sleeping giant in our brains and controls our actions when we are not thinking about it. This is the reason it is important to pay attention to this often neglected part of our mind. It is like an autopilot system. What is great about this system is that once it is set properly, lifestyle change becomes easy because it becomes automatic.

It is like a boat that is going in one direction and you want to change its direction. You could grab the wheel and keep it turned in the new direction. However, if you get tired and let go of the wheel, the boat will resume its old pre-set autopilot direction. This is like behavior change effort that fails all too often. People get tired of the new changes and they give up and old habits take over. How do we change this? We do so by changing the autopilot settings. Once you do that, you can let the wheel go and rest and you will still be going in the right direction.

How to Reset Our Autopilot Habits

So how do we reset our "autopilot"? We do so by repetitive messages to our subconscious. The reason I say "positive" messages, is because our subconscious mind is powerful but simplistic. It responds by moving us towards pictures or images that are presented to it especially when enhanced with color, sound, movement, and all your senses.

For example, when you were young and wanted to learn to ride a bike, and you saw a rock in the road, if you said to yourself, *"Don't hit the rock - don't hit the rock - don't hit the rock!"* What happens? Often you will hit the rock because your subconscious responded to the picture you presented. The image that would work better is, *"Stay on the road - stay on the road - stay on the road!"* and you are more likely to stay on the path you prefer.

In this example, I intentionally repeated the same phrase because repetition is useful in making an impression on the subconscious. This is where self-talk becomes important. We need to control our internal conversation if we want to make the most of our subconscious autopilot system. This is a place where choice of words is very important because it can control the setting of your subconscious and your habitual responses to situations.

Positive affirmations are useful in keeping our thoughts focused and likely to make a positive impression on our subconscious mind. There are some simple rules to use in order to make effective affirmations. To some extent, these rules are there to allow the "law of attraction" to take hold. The law of attraction basically is that what you intentionally picture clearly in your mind repeatedly tends to become reality. This is partly based on setting your autopilot in a positive direction. Here are 7 basic rules - the seven "P's" of making good positive affirmations. They are meant to be repeated to yourself over and over to have a positive influence on your subconscious and engage your subconscious mind in achieving your goals:

7 "P's" for Positive Affirmations

1. Make them Positive: write about what you want - not what you don't want.
2. Make them Powerful: When possible, make them have an emotional impact on you by connecting to something you truly desire, and using devices such as sight, sound, and movement.
3. Make them Personal: It has to be about you and your role and accomplishment.
4. Make them Present: See your outcome as already accomplished.
5. Make them Precise: Set it to specific numbers and dates and vivid detail.
6. Make them Plausible: You must be able to believe in them.
7. Make them Private: Keep it to yourself or within your trusted mastermind group.

Meditation

Meditation has long been acknowledged to have a positive impact on stress and health. There are many types and techniques of meditation. Basically meditation simply means to focus your thoughts in a quiet contemplative way. Meditation is part of every religion, and it can be independent of any religion. It is one way to use your thoughts and mind in a way that can reduce your stress and reduce your risk of heart disease. Meditation can be practiced by anyone.

There are many variations to meditation. For example it can include positive imagery, scripture, breathing, mindfulness, yogic positions, mantras, chanting, emptying the mind or any combination of these aspects. Some of the more popular forms of meditation include Transcendental Meditation, Vipassana Meditation, Zen Meditation, and Mindfulness Meditation, to name a few. Meditation can simply help us to relax. It can also help us reach our subconscious mind and tap into its power including its psychoneuroimmunological effect. If done with techniques with view to opening the mind, it can also be a way to connect with the infinite, and it can be like prayer.

Here is what one of my favorite meditation instructors Dr. Raj Kumar suggests in starting to do meditation. He does suggest that if you want to learn meditation in earnest, you should find a teacher. Meanwhile, you can start with this simple exercise as described in his book "The Secrets of Health and Healing."

Sit comfortably with your eyes closed. Shift your awareness towards your natural breathing. Experience your breath flowing through your nostrils and its effect on your system. Be conscious of the present moment. if your mind starts wandering, know that it is normal .

Do not block or suppress any thoughts; at the same time do not invite any. . . .

After regular practice of meditation, you will get to a point where:

. . . we are capable of experiencing the so-called blank space where thoughts just come and go without affecting our emotions. . . . Express thanks to God.   The mind transcends to a state of selflessness, evoking love, compassion, forgiveness, and positive thinking. In this state, you regain an abunce of energy and wish to utilize it positively.   Raj Kumar

Love

I use the label of Love to describe the importance of our emotions to our health. Three of the most important concepts in this aspect of health are 1) unconditional love, 2) forgiveness, and 3) gratitude. Even as nebulous as these topics may be, there is now scientific literature that confirms that this is important for health.

In Hawaii, we always greet people with "aloha." The true meaning of "aloha" is the sharing of unconditional, universal love and is often lost in the tourist notion that it means "hello" and "goodbye." The literal derivation of the word is the combination of "alo" or "face-to-face" and "ha" which means the "breath of life." So it means "face-to-face, I share with you the breath of life from God." In a sense it means that we are connected through this breath of life.

As so much a part of the spirit of Hawaii and its legacy, we teach "Aloha" at the Center for Attitudinal Healing. We teach that the essence of our being is Love. It is comprised of the idea that you always wake up and go to bed in the spirit of Aloha, meaning you give always unconditional universal love to everyone. My Hanai (adoptive) mother Agnes Kalanihookaha Cope used to say when you greet people, don't forget that you are greeting the spirit of God within them. In other words, we should love everyone because it is a way to love God, and the love will come back to us because we are connected through God. And the more love we give, the more we will get back. That's a great lesson to learn.

It is important to give Love and to give as much as you can. You see, there is an alchemy in giving unconditional love that is greater than any commodity. For example, if you give someone five dollars, you have five dollars less and that person has five dollars more. But if you give love, that person has more love and you also have more love. What s deal! You give something of value to someone and they are richer and in the same transaction, you are richer. Everyone wins! So why not give as much love as you can. It will only make you a richer person. After all, I believe that giving as much love as you can while you are alive is one of the main reasons you were given a life.

The essence of our being is love. Because of this reality, cultivating a spirit of unconditional love for ourselves and others is one of the most important things you can do. You should love yourself and you should love your neighbors as yourself and you should ultimately love God with all your heart, mind, and soul.

If you find that you have trouble with the concepts in this section such as giving, love, forgiving others and yourself, and feeling gratitude, you are not alone. This section which, deals with the emotional side of things, is for some people is the most difficult part of the Peace Diet concept. This is because much of our behavior is based not just on what we eat or think but also on our emotional past. If you find yourself emotionally stuck, you might need some help such as from your pastor, your spiritual advisor or a life coach. My cousin Mari Shintani, who does such coaching says:

> *"Most important for emotional and or physical health is to release all of the negativity and baggage of one's lifetime-the foundation of which begins at the point of origin, so that one is able to move forward in a new and positive direction."* – www.aloha-ai-wellness.com

Forgiveness

The legendary founder of the "Attitudinal Healing" movement, Dr. Jerry Jampolsky wrote a book called "Forgiveness: The Greatest Healer of All." He and his wife, Dr. Diane Cirincione have created an international movement that promotes inner peace and healing through managing our own attitudes. They sometimes quote Buddha as saying "Holding a grudge is like taking poison and hoping the other person will die."

Forgiveness is not always easy, but it generally benefits the forgiver more than the forgiven. And let's face it, none of us is perfect. If we look deeply enough, we will usually find that at one time or another, we have been guilty of what the other person has done to make us angry. This is why it is important to see ourselves in the other person and to forgive ourselves as well.

In his book, Dr. Jampolsky gives a simple example of jogging on the beautiful island of Molokai in Hawaii and being upset about seeing a couple of beer cans littering the side of the road. His first thought was to be judgmental about how inconsiderate this awful person was to litter this beautiful place and he became angry. Then he remembered how he himself when he was younger at times had tossed trash out of his car window. He then decided to pick up the beer cans and felt not only forgiving and releasing the other person from his judgment but also releasing himself of his own guilt.

Dr. Jampolsky hastens to point out that it didn't mean he agreed with or condoned what the other person had done. It simply meant that he freed himself from the aggravation of his own judgmental thoughts and feelings. Dr. Cirincione also points out that it is important to separate the act from the person. One may dislike bad acts or outcomes but one should always love people. In other words, never allow yourself to hate others. You can hate the actions and what happens but don't hate the people. If you do, in the end, some of it will come back to you. And in the same way, if you give love - as much as you can, that will also eventually come back to you.

THE 12 PRINCIPLES OF ATTITUDINAL HEALING

1. The essence of our being is love.
2. Health is inner peace. Healing is letting go of fear.
3. Giving and receiving are the same.
4. We can let go of the past and the future.
5. Now is the only time there is and each instant is for giving.
6. We can learn to love ourselves and others by forgiving rather than judging.
7. We can become love finders rather than fault finders.
8. We can choose and direct ourselves to be peaceful inside regardless of what is happening outside.
9. We are students and teachers to each other.
10. We can focus on the whole of life rather than the fragments.
11. Since love is eternal death need not be viewed as fearful.
12. We can always perceive ourselves and others as either extending love or giving a call for help.

For a full explanation of these principles go to the website of Attitudinal Healing International at www.ahinternational.org and also go the website of the Hawaii Center for Attitudinal Healing at www.ahhawaii.org. There are resources there including video interviews explaining these 12 Principles of Attitudinal healing. There are also support group sessions and training sessions that you may be able to access through these websites.

Gratitude

Scientific research shows that gratitude is healing.[85, 86, 87, 88]

Like love and forgiveness, giving thanks and holding an attitude of gratitude costs us nothing but pays great dividends.

Here is a list of some of the reported benefits of gratitude. According to research, people who have gratitude wind up having the following benefits. They:

- Take better care of themselves
- Eat better
- Exercise more
- Are more alert mentally
- Feel happier
- Have fewer physical complaints
- Handle stress better
- Have a stronger immune function.

Based on this research, it's a good idea to make it a habit of making a list of things for which we are grateful and review it every day.

Here is a poem about gratitude written by my teacher Michio Kushi in his book, "The Book of Macrobiotics" that I think expresses the spirit of gratitude. It is worthy of repeating daily if you can't come up with your own list of things you are grateful for.

I am grateful to my parents and ancestors,
I am grateful to my spouse and partner,
I am grateful to my children and offspring,
I am grateful to all people and all beings,

I am grateful to the foods I am given,
I am grateful to the nature that I am within,
I am grateful to the universe in which I am manifested,
I am grateful to all phenomena and all beings,

I am grateful to my sickness,
I am grateful to my ignorance,
I am grateful to my enemy,
I am grateful to my difficulties,
I am grateful to my suffering,

I am nothing, yet I have been given all,
Therefore, I am rich, equal to the whole universe.
I am endlessly grateful to my being here and now.
Michio Kushi 1984

In the book in which this is written, "The Book of Macrobiotics" this poem is called a "prayer." Of course, poems can be used as prayers. In the next section we discuss the importance of prayer in our pursuit of health and peace.

Prayer

I believe that we are not just physical beings. We are spiritual beings as well. After all, the Holy Bible says, "in the beginning, God created the heavens AND the earth," not just the earth. So there is a spiritual world as well as the physical world. I believe all healing comes from God, often called "The Great Physician." Because of this, our relationship with God, is important to acknowledge. It is the great mystery of every living thing - how we were given the breath of life, how our bodies perform such complex things as converting food to energy, and how our bodies heal themselves. This is why every time I conduct a program, I always start with a prayer.

If you are not religiously inclined, you can feel a connection to a higher being and a spiritual component through the universal consciousness that we are all part of a greater universe. Think about it. Life is not just a physical entity with a bunch of chemicals wrapped up in a bag of skin. At the moment just before death and just after the chemicals in the body are essentially the same. But what has changed? The answer is the spirit has left the body. If you have trouble believing that there is a spirit, consider the evidence of near-death experiences.

One unforgettable account described in a book "Life at Death" by Dr. Kenneth Ring, was about a patient who had essentially died on the operating table and her doctors were able to revive her. When she woke up, she described how she began to rise out of her body and up through the ceiling of the hospital. As she hovered above the hospital, she saw a red shoe on the roof. Then, as she was being revived, she was pulled back into her body. When the doctor heard this story, he sent a maintenance man to see what was on the roof and when he came back, in his hand was a red shoe.

One of my teachers, affectionately called the "Cosmic Dancer" was my religion professor, Rev. Mits Aoki. He had a life-changing experience when he died in an auto accident, and was brought back by the Emergency Medical Tech's. While his heart had apparently stopped, he recalled floating above the scene and seeing himself being resuscitated. The experience was a life-changing experience and he quit his ministry and became a professor of religion to teach students about his new perspective in a course called "The Meaning of Existence." There are numerous stories such as this that validate the existence of a spiritual component to life. To acknowledge and enhance the spiritual side of life, I consider prayer as one of the most important things you can do to support your health.

My Experience with Prayer

When I was 6 months old in 1951, my father was diagnosed with colon cancer. They took out the whole left side of his colon and left him with a permanent colostomy. They said he would be lucky to live another couple of years. My father had a second surgery when I was just 3 years old, and I remember feeling afraid of losing him. Imagine what it's like for a 3-year-old to understand the meaning of the word "metastasis" (the spreading of cancer)?

So I began to pray - every night. *"Dear God. Please don't let Dad die of cancer. . ."* Every single night I prayed that simple prayer - for years - decades. Fortunately, he lived another 40 years and never died of cancer. I will always believe that my prayers had something to do with his survival. After all, how many people do you know of who survived colon cancer in the 1950's? I will always believe that prayer contributed to saving my father's life.

I have also looked to prayer for guidance. For me, it is a way to communicate with the Almighty. I ask for guidance when I am faced with difficult decisions. In my opinion, there are two general types of prayer. For lack of a better way to categorize it, I see prayer as either "yin" prayer, - expanding to the universe and in praise of God, and "yang" prayer in which we ask for assistance from God to manifest an outcome on Earth.

I am sometimes asked 'what is the difference between meditation and prayer?'. In my opinion, there is some overlap. Meditation can be prayerful, and prayer can be meditative. However, I believe that fundamentally, meditation reaches inside us to the power of our subconscious and the great power within us. If done properly, however, meditation can also connect us to the infinite and tap into an intelligence outside of us such that we can "hear the voice of God", and if we begin to communicate with that voice, then it becomes like prayer. Prayer is a way to reach outside of us to a power beyond us - to the infinite to the Almighty for guidance, strength, and help.

In a way, the difference is something like the way a computer works. It is as if the conscious mind is the computer's RAM memory (these days about 4 gigabytes) and the subconscious is the hard drive - (around 500 gigabytes). So meditation to reach the subconscious is very powerful. But prayer is like reaching the internet - all knowing and all seeing and so much more powerful with access to billions of websites and computers around the world.

In a similar way, prayer can access resources beyond you. There is no power greater than being in sync with the Almighty. So always remember the power of the spirit, and the power of prayer when you need guidance, when you need strength and when you need healing.

A 3-Minute Daily Routine for Optimal Health

In order to incorporate these aspects of health in your life, I suggest a 7-Item daily routine to be done every morning and every night before bed. I suggest a 3-minute routine that includes the following just after arising and just before going to bed. The reason for this timing is simple. First, you are much less likely to forget if it is a routine that you do daily at a time that provides a cue for you to remember - like going to bed or waking up in the morning. Second, your mind is closer to alpha rhythm which helps you to meditate and to make an impression on your subconscious with the lists in your daily routine.

First, make 5 lists before you go to bed. This should take longer than 3 minutes at first but as you begin to do this regularly, the time may be condensed down to about 3 minutes or so although, if you have more time that would be even better. The five lists include:
1. Plan for your meals -
2. Plan for your exercise - make an appointment with yourself
3. Plan for your work - your to-do list
4. Plan for your love - your to-be list (how you will give love to others)
5. Your affirmations.

The daily routine should be timed something like this.

The 7 Steps Daily Routine

1. 15 sec. Review your plan for your healthy meals
2. 15 sec. Review your plan for your exercise - make an appointment with yourself.
3. 15 sec. Review your "to-do" list
4. 15 sec. Review your "to-be" list (how you will "be" and give love to others)
5. 30 sec. Declare your affirmations
6. 30 sec. Meditate - relax, visualize
7. 1 min. Pray

This will help you stay on track with your diet and exercise. It can also bring into play the power of your mind, body and spirit by having you not only follow the Peace Diet menu but also bring into play the power of the 4 intentions that surround the Peace Diet diagram - the power of exercise, of thoughts, of love and of prayer.

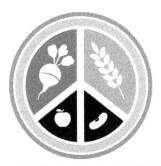

VII- GETTING STARTED WITH THE PEACE DIET

To begin, I suggest that every evening and every morning you do a simple, 3-minute exercise described above covering the 7 basic components of the Peace Diet, to make yourself familiar with the other, non-food mealtime and lifestyle activities that put you on the path to optimal health. Let this time be a meditative time, and remember that the Peace Diet is inspired by the eating patterns of those who were seeking spiritual health.

When you understand its foundations, getting started making Peace Diet meals is quite simple, as it is based on long-standing traditional practices. The diet's signature Peace Plate gives simple guidance as to the proportions of each of its food groups and which types of food to consume, to assist you with planning your meals.

When I myself got started on it, I learned how to make just four simple things:

- Whole grains
- Stir-fried vegetables
- Simple bean dishes
- Soup

Grains

Grains have been the center of the traditional diets of virtually every great civilization on earth. The most commonly consumed grain in the world is rice, and the very first cooking skill I learned was how to make brown rice—a useful skill, since most all other whole grains are cooked in a similar way. The best way is to cook your grains is in a stainless steel pressure cooker (be careful never to use aluminum pressure cookers).

It is helpful to add a pinch of salt at the beginning for each cup of rice being cooked. Pressure- cooking is faster than simple boiling and keeps the nutrients and flavor in the food. An automatic rice cooker also makes things very simple, although I don't consider this appliance as useful as a pressure-cooker, because of the way it allows steam and nutrients to escape.

If you don't have either of these appliances, read the directions in the recipe section below for guidelines on how to cook rice in a stainless steel pot. I like to use basmati brown rice because it has a nice fragrance and a nutty aroma. If you want your rice to be a little fancier, you can throw in a handful of wheat berries to give the dish a little bit of color and texture, or you could also go to a health food market and look over the selection of boxed kits that are available for purchase; there are pre-mixed spice kits for rice dishes which include such flavors as mushroom rice, Spanish rice, lentil-and-rice combinations, and so forth.

Vegetables

A vegetable stir-fry is terrifically versatile, and also quite a simple dish to learn. When I myself was first learning to make these dishes, I had to first learn how to go about cutting up the vegetables I wanted in the stir-fry into shapes and sizes that would cook properly and not become mushy, soggy, or burned. Nowadays I usually start with onions, cutting them vertically so the pieces are crescent-shaped instead of round rings, which helps them to stay crisp. Then I chop up my more solid vegetables such as broccoli, carrots, cauliflower, and zucchini. More delicate vegetables, such as cabbage, kale, collards, won bok, watercress, and mung bean sprouts cook most quickly, and are added last.

I start by sautéing the onions first until they are translucent, in a little bit of extra-virgin olive oil or vegetable broth. Thicker vegetables, like broccoli, go in next, and the quicker-cooking, leafier vegetables or sprouts are added to the pan last. Stir fry for another few minutes at medium heat and then turn off the stove and cover the pan to allow the vegetables to steam themselves. You can judge the time so that its texture meets with your satisfaction.

As I stir-fry the vegetables, instead of adding more oil, I use vegetable broth as needed. To add flavor, I might also add a few dashes of soy sauce, or Bragg's Liquid Aminos which is a low-sodium organic substitute for soy sauce sold at health-food stores. Before the vegetables are cooked crisp-tender I cover the wok with a lid, to let the vegetables steam. For variety, I vary the vegetables. Leftovers make a great vegetarian wrap when rolled up into a whole-wheat tortilla.

In addition to cooked vegetable dishes, salads are also easy to make, and raw vegetables are also important to include in your diet. Raw vegetables are harder to digest because they are naturally protected by surface coverings, much of which is insoluble fiber such as cellulose. Because of this, it's important to chew your vegetables well, so that you make all the nutrients in them available to your body. For salad dressings, it's important to use no-oil dressings, or the dressings that have the least amount of fat or oil in them; remember, most vegetable oils have lots of those omega-6 fatty acids that can promote inflammation, raise cholesterol, and carry lots of calories.

Beans

Bean dishes are especially simple to prepare by using pre-cooked canned beans. I myself really like black beans, which can be prepared very simply by adding a little salt, chili powder, onion powder, and some soy or barbecue sauce. The basic recipe is easy: mix the ingredients, heat, and stir. It's simple because the beans are already cooked.

Tofu, made of soybeans, is another simple bean-based meal option. It can be eaten cold with soy sauce, or cooked in any dish for which you might have used meat or chicken. One of the most appealing dishes I learned is called "tofu nuggets." Never tried tofu? Don't knock it 'til you've tried it! Even kids want second helpings of this savory dish.

Soup

One of the best things about soup is that you can put one, two, or three categories of Peace Diet foods into one dish. Miso, an ingredient made from fermented soybean paste, makes one of my favorite soup recipes, a traditional Japanese soup base that has served Asian chefs well for centuries. Miso soup is extremely simple because the miso itself does not have to be cooked - you just add the miso paste at the end into the hot water and everything else you put into your soup tastes great. It's as easy as instant soup in a cup!

The trick to this deliciously robust, nourishing soup is to find a good source of miso. Today it is quite common in health food stores, but you can also find various types of it in Oriental food stores. In a supermarket without an Oriental foods section miso may be more difficult to find, but if you ask the manager, he or she will often be able to order it for you.

Simply prepare some of your favorite vegetables such as mushrooms, broccoli, carrots, and cabbage in boiling water, then, just before serving, dissolve some miso paste in it as described in the recipe below, and blend smoothly make sure any lumps are removed. For variety, you can add cooked barley or similar grains to the mixture. Miso is very high in protein and is a great substitute for any animal product-based soup, but it is also quite high in sodium; this, though, can be controlled by the amount of miso you use.

Fruit

Few people need to learn how to prepare fruit, which is always best eaten fresh and in season. It needs no preparation, except for washing, though there are recipes for cooked fruit if you have a festive occasion. The most popular of these is apple crisp, which tastes like apple pie, but without the white flour crust.

Making the Peace Diet Your Own

The simple dishes described above are how I got started preparing healthful meals for myself and are examples of the ones used in my programs. There are sample menus and recipes in the next chapter, to accommodate your own tastes. Feel free to experiment and try new things. As you begin the Peace Diet, remember that your tastes will change because as you begin to eat healthier food, your taste buds and your cravings will adjust. Most people find that the highly-salted, sugary, greasy foods they may have enjoyed in the past become unpleasant, or, if returned to, create uncomfortable sensations afterwards. This makes it much easier to stay with the Peace Diet!

RECIPES

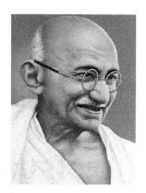

"The greatness of a nation and its moral progress can be judged by the way its animals are treated."

"To my mind, the life of a lamb is no less precious than that of a human being."

Mahatma Gandhi, statesman and philosopher (1869-1948)

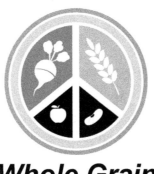

Whole Grain

Grains have been a major food source in many areas of the world throughout history, and for good reason. They're loaded with protein, fiber, vitamins, and minerals. They are inexpensive to buy and easy to cook with. You can use them in soups, salads, side dishes, and main dishes. They are delicious in everything from breakfast cereals 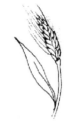 to pasta, to bread and even in desserts. The key is to be sure that you're using whole grains, not refined grains. Refined grains such as those found in white flour and white rice cause grains to be stripped of fiber and nutrients, but using whole grains is beneficial even to the point of reducing the risk of diabetes, heart disease, stroke, and cancer.

Whole grains provide both soluble and insoluble fiber. Soluble fiber lowers blood cholesterol, while insoluble fiber prevents constipation and can help protect against certain cancers. Whole grains are also beneficial by creating a feeling of fullness, which can help dieters to eat less.

There are hundreds of different grains. In the list below I've chosen common varieties that you will easily find in your supermarket or health food store. Remember to store all grains in a cool, dry place to retain longest shelf life (which can be months).

Easy Cooking, Lots of Uses

Often people avoid cooking with whole grains because they're not sure how to prepare them, but the chart below demonstrates that it's fairly easy. Always try to keep grains as close to their natural state as possible. Here are some fast, easy recipes to get you started.

Cooking Chart for Grains

Regular Pot			Pressure Cooker	
1 Cup of Grain	Cups Water	Time	Cups Water	Time
Rolled Oats	2-2.5*	20-25 min.	n/a	n/a
Brown Rice	2	40-55 min.	1.5-1.75	30-40 min.
Buckwheat	2-2.5*	2-2.5 hrs.	n/a	n/a
Pearled Barley	2	25-30 min.	1.25	15 min.
Hulled Barley	2.5-3*	1.5-1.75 hrs.	2.5	20-25 min.
Bulgur Wheat	1.5-2*	20 min.	n/a	n/a
Whole Wheat	2	1.5-2 hrs.	1.5	20-25 min.
Oats, Rye	2	1-2 hrs.	1.5	20-25 min.
Millet	2	25-35 min.	1.5	15 min.

*Lower number will yield a slightly chewier grain.
Higher   number   will   yield   a   slightly   softer   grain.

Rice Dishes

More people eat rice worldwide than any other single food. Rice is rich in beneficial complex carbohydrates, low in fat and calories, and rich in nutrients when it has not been refined. Rice aids digestion and has been found to assist in lowering the risk for diabetes, obesity, high cholesterol, and heart disease.

Brown rice is the most nutritious form of rice and the only one that contains vitamin E. This is because only the inedible husk has been removed. It is full of satisfying complex carbohydrates, fiber, B complex vitamins, and other nutrients. It has a nutty flavor and chewy texture; it takes slightly longer to cook than white rice. Brown rice comes in many varieties: long grain, short grain, and medium grain. You can choose from basmati rice, jasmine rice, arborio, plain brown, Thai black, long grain wild rice, and risotto. Here are some characteristics of just a few of the varieties:

- Basmati rice is very fragrant, comes from India and Pakistan, and doubled in length when it's cooked. It can be substituted for regular rice in most recipes.
- Arborio rice is creamy white rice grown in Italy and often used for classic Italian risotto dishes. It can also be used in paella and rice pudding.
- Jasmine rice was originally from Thailand but is now grown in the United States. It is similar to basmati and good in Southeast Asian dishes.

For delicious, easy-to-prepare dishes, experiment with some of these varieties to find out which ones appeal most to you. But remember to choose brown rice or the darker varieties since they have the most nutrition.

Ah, Technology!

Cooking rice and other grains has become easier -- basically foolproof! Automatic rice cookers are a great aid because they turn themselves off automatically when the rice is cooked. All you have to do is put in the proper amount of water. These cookers do a good job of steaming rice as well. Foolproof directions are included with the appliance.

Rice-Cooker Rice

Ratio:
2C   Water
1C   Brown rice
      pinch Sea salt

Wash and rinse rice, add the water and turn on the cooker. Adjust the water to your liking. (See appliance instructions for cooking times.) Makes 2 portions. (1 portion = 216 calories, 1.8 grams fat, 9% protein, 83% carbohydrates, 7% fat). '

Gourmet Rice Is a Breeze

What's better than eating "gourmet" food that's been easy, breezy to prepare? Not much! That's what you can have when you prepare basmati brown rice. Basmati is known as the "King of Rice." Originating in India, it's been enjoyed by their elite for centuries. It's rich and aromatic and is enjoyed by almost everyone who tries it (it's my personal favorite). Easy to find and easy to prepare, cook it like any other brown rice.

Basmati Brown Rice

2C   Basmati (or other brown Rice)
3½-4 C   Water
2 pinches   Sea salt

Gently wash rice until water rinses clear. If possible, soak for 2 to 6 hours.

Place in 2-quart pot (stainless steel is best). Cover rice with water and add sea salt. Cover, bring to a boil, reduce flame then simmer for 45 minutes to one hour. (Do not uncover rice while cooking.) When done, remove from flame and let sit for 10 more minutes before serving.

Makes 6 cup portions. (1 portion = 216 calories, 1.8 grams fat, 9% protein, 83% carbohydrates, 7% fat)

Kitchari - An Ayurvedic Weight-Loss and Detox Dish

A simple variation on Basmati rice makes it into "kitchari" which is a popular ayurvedic health dish. Some people will eat just kitchari for several days to do a dietary cleanse or detox. "Kitchari" simply means "mixture". For this dish, it is mainly a mixture of Basmati rice with mung beans and some spices. Here is a simple recipe and also a list of ingredients to make it more elaborate.

Simple Kitchari

1cup	basmati rice
1 cup	yellow split mung dal
1/2 tsp	turmeric
1 small	handful cilantro leaves, chopped
6 cups	water
	Sea salt and pepper to taste.

Wash the rice and mung dal twice, using plenty of water. If you have time, let the mung dal soak for a few hours before cooking, to help with digestibility.

Add rice, dal, turmeric and cilantro to the water. Bring to a boil, and boil 5 minutes uncovered, stirring occasionally.

Turn down heat to low, and cover, leaving the lid slightly ajar. Cook until tender, about 25 to 30 minutes. Season with salt and pepper to taste.

Here are additional optional seasonings to add with the turmeric f you have time and the ingredients.

1/4 teaspoon mustard seeds
1 1/2 teaspoons cumin
1 teaspoon fenugreek

1. tsp fennel

1 tsp coriander powder
1 tsp fresh ginger

1 pinch Hing (acefetida)

Effortless Options

Another good thing about whole grains is their flexibility. You can vary the overall taste effortlessly by adding other types of grains to your brown rice. Then add in some vegetables and top off with some sauces or gravies. All your choices can be both nutritious and delicious. The variations are endless, depending on your imagination and taste.

Here are two suggestions, just to get you started:

- Add in some wild rice. This rice came from the seed of a swamp grass and in the past grew only in the wild, but now it is also cultivated. It has an interesting woodsy flavor and is packed with iron, protein, niacin and fiber.
- How about wheat berries? Wheat berries are whole, unprocessed kernels of wheat, so they are loaded with nutrients and fiber. They are chewy and have a subtle, nutty flavor.

Popular, Versatile Pilafs

You're probably familiar with some type of rice pilaf dish, but did you know that rice pilaf was originally a Persian dish containing rice, raisins, meats or fowl, and a sauce? These days, pilafs are a part of the cuisine all over the world. There's Spanish Rice Pilaf, Indian Saffron Rice Pilaf, and American Lentil Rice, to name only a few. Making rice pilaf is another way to easily please by presenting "gourmet" meals with little effort on your part. The trick once again is to add some chopped vegetables and spices and condiments to the rice. It's a small effort that obtains a great result.

These delicious pilaf recipes will give you some ideas, but do join in the fun and create your own. Lack of time does not need to be a problem. You can even try prepackaged pilaf mixes minus the oil and butter...very convenient.

Stovetop Rice Pilaf

1/8 C	Mild yellow onion, finely chopped
1/8 C	Green onion or shallot, finely chopped
1/8 C	Celery, chopped (about ¼" pieces)
½C	Carrots, julienned
½C	Vegetable broth
1C	Brown rice, presteamed till fluffy (see Tip #6)
½C	Wheat berries, presteamed with rice
	Black ground pepper, 1/8 tsp.

In a large, non-stick skillet, sauté onion in 2 tablespoons of vegetable broth until tender. Add remaining vegetable broth, heat, then add other ingredients (except celery) and sauté, stirring constantly, until carrots are hot through and slightly tender (about 5 minutes). Add celery to skillet at the very end, leaving a lot of crunch to the celery. Add precooked rice and wheat berries to the skillet mixture, mix well while cooking a few more minutes, to blend the flavors. Fluff and serve. Makes 5 portions. (1 portion = 76.3
calories, 0.5 grams fat, 12% protein, 83% carbohydrates, 5% fat) Wheat berries take longer to cook than does the rice, so should come out softened but still crunchy. Pilafs and stir-fries are best when they offer a variety of textures.

Baked Wild Rice Pilaf

3C	Vegetable broth or konbu broth
1 med.	Mild yellow onion, diced (about ¼ to 1/3 cup)
3 cloves	Garlic, minced
1 stalk	Celery, diced (about ½ cup)
1½ C	Fresh mushrooms, thinly sliced
1C	Wild rice
1½ tsp.	Tamari
½ tsp.	Sesame seeds, Toasted
	pinch Sea salt

To make konbu broth, soak one 3" x 3" piece of konbu in mineral water for 1 hour.   In a nonstick skillet, sauté onions, garlic, celery, and mushrooms in a little vegetable broth until onions are translucent. Add water only if this mixture begins to stick to pan, though it shouldn't if you stir constantly and turn to medium heat. In a saucepan, bring konbu stock to a boil. Pour into skillet with other ingredients, mix well, then place all in a casserole or baking dish. Cover and bake at 350o F. for 1½ hours. Remove cover and bake another 15 to 20 minutes to remove any excess liquid. Makes 3 portions. (1 portion = 264.9 calories, 1.3 grams fat, 20% protein, 76% carbohydrates, 4% fat)

Serve with a leafy green salad, for a well- rounded meal. ▽

Stovetop Spanish Rice

1 can	Whole tomatoes, stewed (15 oz.)
½C	Green pepper, diced
1C	Water
¾C	Vegetable broth
¾C	Brown rice, Uncooked
½ tsp.	Sea salt
2 tsp.	Chili powder (or to taste)

Combine tomatoes, pepper, water, salt, and chili powder in medium saucepan. Boil over medium heat. Add rice.

Reduce heat to low, cover, and simmer most of the liquid has been absorbed, about 45 minutes

Fluff rice, replace cover, and let stand 5 minutes before serving. Makes 4 portions. (1 portion = 174.1 calories, 1.5 grams fat, 11% protein, 82% carbohydrates, 7% fat). You may also garnish this dish with finely diced uncooked tomatoes and green pepper, for extra texture and fresh taste. To be really creative, add a tiny bit of chopped fresh cilantro to the top of your served mounds of rice.

Quinoa Pilaf

½C	Mushrooms, sliced
½C	Onion, finely chopped
2C	Vegetable broth
1C	Quinoa, toasted (see below)
½C	Celery, chopped
½C	(about ½" segments) Carrot, shredded
1/3 C	Green bell pepper, finely chopped Red bell pepper,
1/3 C	finely chopped Yellow bell pepper, finely chopped
1/3 C	Sea salt, to taste dash

Rinse thoroughly

Toasted Quinoa: under cool running water. Place in a 10" to 12" skillet over medium heat; cook, shaking pan occasionally, until quinoa dries and turns golden brown, about 15 minutes. Pour toasted quinoa from pan and let cool. Makes 1 cup. Water-sauté onions and mushrooms in a large (10" to 12") skillet over medium heat, until onions are caramelized and mushrooms are golden brown. To water sauté, simply put a few tablespoons of water in a skillet, let it heat, then add onions and mushrooms. Stir often. If it begins to stick, add a bit more water. Add broth, quinoa, and allvegetables, bring to a boil, lower heat, cover then simmer until liquid is absorbed, about 15 minutes, stirring often. *Makes 6 portions. (1 portion = 133.6 calories, 1.8 grams fat, 17% protein, 72% carbohydrates, 12% fat).*

Vegetarian Eight Treasures

This is a great traditional Chinese dish that was used by the legendary Shaolin Monks to support their health, strength and spiritual development.

2	Bean curd or tofu cakes
1 tsp.	Peanut oil
1 medium	Cucumber
1 medium	Carrot
4	dried shiitake mushrooms
1 can	Water chestnuts
1/2 lb.	Chinese peas
2 tsp.	Chili paste
2 Tbsp.	miso
3 Tbsp.	Soy sauce
1-1/2 Tbsp.	Sugar
1 Tbsp.	Rice wine
1-1/2 Tbsp.	Water
1/4 C	Peanuts, unsalted and dry roasted

Soak bean curd in hot water for one hour. Drain by placing bean curd between paper towels. Place a light weight on wrapped bean curd for 1 hour. Cut into 1/2" pieces.

Soak the mushrooms in water and cut into 1/2" pieces

Dice the cucumber and carrots in 1/2" pieces. Steam for 8 minutes.

Drain and dice water chestnuts.

In a skillet or wok water-sauté carrot, water chestnuts, bean curd, peas, mushrooms and cucumber for 1 to 2 minutes. Remove from skillet or wok.

In the same pan, stir fry peanut oil and chili paste for about 10 seconds. Add miso and soy sauces, sugar, rice wine, and water until sauce begins to thicken. Add the cooked vegetables and peanuts and toss lightly until mixed. Serve. *Most of the fat in this recipe comes from the peanuts and peanut oil, so go easy on them to keep the fat content down.*

Makes 6 portions. *(1 portion = 142 calories, 5.6 grams fat, 21% protein, 44% carbohydrates, 34% fat).*

Healthy Breakfast Alternative

We love breakfast cereals, and oatmeal or whole grain cereals are a good way to start the day. It's the milk and/or sugar we add that make breakfast less healthy for reasons we've discussed. But there's a way to enjoy whole grain cereal without sugar and dairy…and it can still be enjoyable. Simply dry-roast the grains in a hot skillet before you cook them in water. This process ("dextrinizing") will make your meal delicious. Often, simple tips like this one lead to delicious breakfasts.

Dry-roasting your grain before you cook it will give it a rich, nutty flavor.

Toasty Cooked Breakfast Cereal

1C Dry oatmeal, bulgur wheat or other breakfast whole grain.

Dry-roast grains by putting them in a nonstick skillet. Roast over a low flame or heat, shaking and tossing a little until it browns and a nice toasty aroma rises out of the pan. Then prepare as you would ordinarily.

Gandule Rice

This is a dish that everyone should try at least once. It is a Puerto Rican dish that is very low in fat and has a zesty flavor. It was probably the best liked recipe in our cooking classes.

4C	Rice, uncooked, washed, and drained
2C	Gandule beans or 1 can gandule beans (15 oz.), drained
1	Bell pepper, chopped
1	large Onion, diced
2 bunches	Cilantro, chopped
3-4 cloves	Garlic
2-3 stalks	Celery, diced
1 can	Tomato sauce (8 oz.)
1 env	Goya powder or chili powder
	Salt, to taste or Vegesol®
1 tsp.	Cumin
1 tsp.	Oregano
1-2 tsp.	Extra virgin olive oil
3C	Vegetarian chicken-flavored broth
	Olives, sliced
	Chinese parsley

In a large pot, sauté all vegetables in olive oil. Add seasonings, goya powder. Add gandules and sauté for another 5 minutes. Add broth and tomato sauce and bring to a boil. Taste and add more salt or seasoning if needed.

Reduce heat to low and simmer for around 35 to 40 minutes or until water is gone and rice is at the desired texture.

Another Versatile Crowd Pleaser

Many of us are accustomed to seeing sweet potatoes at our Thanksgiving feasts, But this family staple, steamed or mashed, because of its delicious taste and pleasing, comfort-food texture can be welcome at any meal. The sweet potato happens to be a nutrition giant as well as a crowd pleaser. It's an excellent source of vitamins C, E, the B vitamins, and high in fiber while extremely low in fat.

Sweet potatoes work well as side dishes or snacks. Try substituting three sweet potato slices for three cookies and save seven grams of fat! If you have a sweet tooth, sweet potatoes are your friend. They are filling and satisfy your sweet tooth without ruining your diet.

Steamed Sweet Potatoes or Yams

6 med.   Sweet potatoes or yams
                           Water

Place whole sweet potatoes in steamer with 1" of water and
steam for approximately 15 minutes or until fork tender. Slice
and serve. Or create glazed sweet potatoes by covering with the
following sauce and baking for 5 more minutes. Makes 6
portions. (1 sweet potato portion = 117.0 calories, 0.125 grams
fat, 7% protein, 93% carbohydrates, 1% fat) (1 yam portion =
127.8 calories, 0.1 grams fat, 5% protein, 94% carbohydrates, 1%
fat)

▽   Sweet potatoes and yams are simple and simply delicious
by themselves. They are great at any meal or as snacks.

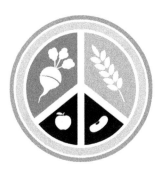

VEGETABLES

Vegetables are nutrition powerhouses; thus, they are essential to the Peace Diet. It's no accident that there's an abundance of wonderful vegetable recipes in this book. Vegetables have the highest rating on the SMI scale, and you should try to eat at least seven to eleven servings per day. Fresh vegetables have the highest nutritive value, followed by frozen and finally by canned.

Both raw and cooked vegetables have nutritional strong points, so it's to your benefit to use both. Using both raw and cooked vegetables gives you not only better protection but also variety. Raw vegetables and juices are recognized around the world not just for their nutritional value but also for their curative value. It is widely believed that five servings of fruits and vegetables per day are associated with lower risk of stroke, obesity and obesity-related diseases, and even aging and degenerative diseases.

Our recipes will cover cooked, raw, and soup vegetables. First, let's take a look at cooked vegetables.

Less Oil, Better Nutrition

A valuable tip is to avoid cooking with oil to whatever extent possible, which is most of the time. For instance, a one-cup serving of vegetables sautéed in oil can have as much as 42% of the calories from fat – which greatly diminishes the overall nutritional value of the dish. This isn't necessary since other ways of cooking work as well and can offer just as much flavor. One way is to use a nonstick ceramic skillet and sauté with water. For more flavor, sauté with canned vegetable broth or a vegetarian powder and water mix.

For more flavor, you can sauté with a little wine or try sautéing a small amount of onion and garlic in the vegetable broth before you add the other ingredients. You will never miss the oil, but you will reap the benefits.

Vegetable Stir Fry

1 can	Mushrooms or ¼ cup dry shiitake mushrooms, soaked and sliced
1 med.	Carrot, sliced diagonally
2 stalks	Broccoli, diagonally sliced
2 stalks	Celery, Diagonally sliced
1½	Round onion, sliced into thin crescents
1 piece	Ginger, crushed
1 clove	Garlic, crushed
1½ Tbsp.	Corn starch
¼C	Water

Seasoning:

1 Tbsp.	Oyster	sauce (vegetarian)
1 tsp.	Soy sauce	
1C	Stock	

Heat pan. Sauté ginger, garlic, and onion in water, remove from pan. Add seasonings and cook 2 minutes. Add stock, mushrooms, carrot, broccoli, and celery and cook until vegetables are crisp and tender. Make a paste with corn starch and water to thicken the gravy. Makes 4 to 6 portions. (1 portion = 59.4 calories, 0.3 grams fat, 19% protein, 77% carbohydrates, 5% fat)

Vegetable Wraps and Mushu Vegetable

Becoming increasingly popular are versatile variations on the vegetable stir fry. Take the leftover stir fry and wrap it in a whole wheat tortilla or chapati (Indian flatbread). For example, you could take leftovers from a stir-fry dinner and in the morning pack a lunch along with some whole wheat tortillas (preferably stone-ground or sprouted grain). Then, at lunch, simply wrap the vegetables in the tortilla - flavor it with soy sauce, barbecue sauce, or any stir-fry sauce of your choice and you have an excellent simple lunch.

As a variation, you can use Hoisin sauce which you can buy where they sell Chinese condiments. This sauce is the secret to a delicious dish usually served at Northern Chinese restaurants called "mushu pork." Of course there is no pork in this dish and it is not necessary. Spreading a thin layer of hoisin sauce makes for a delectable northern Asian dish that you can call "Mushu Vegetable."

Vegetable Side Dishes

Vegetable side dishes should be an important part of your Peace Diet. Steamed vegetables are easy to prepare and are a versatile way to add taste, healthfulness and color to your meal. There are several techniques for steaming, including a bamboo basket over boiling water, a metal steamer over boiling water, or a modern electric steamer that is compact, low cost, has a timer, and makes your steaming foolproof.   Vegetables can also be baked or sautéed depending on the type of vegetable. Whatever form your vegetables take, they are surprisingly rich in nutrients. Here's some information about a few vegetables;   it's fairly representative of the nutrient value of vegetables in general:

- Cauliflower – This cruciferous vegetable, popular for the way it blends and enhances the food it is cooked with, is very high in vitamin C but extremely low in calories and has no fat.
- Broccoli – Another cruciferous vegetable, broccoli is so versatile it can be used in salads, side dishes, soups, stir-frys, or dips. It enhances the other ingredients it is served with, while providing vitamin A, C, calcium, fiber, phytonutrients, and very low calories.
- Carrots – This vegetable may be taken for granted, but it is packed with vitamin A (betacarotene), which is so good for the eyes. Its soluble fiber is good for cholesterol as well.

Some steamed vegetables such as cauliflower, broccoli, julienned carrots, zucchini squash, and so on, are especially good with dipping sauces. These same vegetables may be sliced and used raw, too. Use the sauces above to dip them in, experiment with a variety of them. You'll find that turning your vegetable dishes into wholesome easy snacks - whether raw or steamed - is one of the easiest ways for you to get your several servings of vegetables per day. Try sauces to give your vegetables variety. You'll find several sauces in the Kebab section (p. 173) of these recipes. You can also try the salad dressings for dips as well.

Spicy Szechuan Eggplant

1½ lbs.	Eggplant, peeled and cut into 3" strips
1C	Chinese wood ear fungus (or shiitake straw, or other mushrooms), soaked and sliced into strips
	Canola oil cooking spray
	Garlic Sauce:

¼C	Soy sauce
1 Tbsp.	Honey
1 Tbsp.	Distilled white vinegar
1 Tbsp.	Corn starch
2	red Chili Peppers, minced
2 slices	Ginger, minced
2 cloves	Garlic, minced

Mix all sauce ingredients and set aside.

Spray pan with oil. Sauté eggplant over medium flame until golden brown, about 5 minutes. Combine sauce for 1 minute with eggplant and fungus. Makes 4 portions.

(1 portion = 148 calories, 1.0 grams fat, 15% protein, 79% carbohydrates, 5% fat)

Melt-In-Your-Mouth Kabocha Squash

1   Kabocha or acorn squash

Cut the kabocha squash into 4" squares or cleaned acorn squash in quarters. Place on a baking pan with a tiny bit of water and bake at 350o F. until tender (about an hour). Makes 2 portions. (1 portion = 115.0 calories, 0.290 grams fat, 7% protein, 91% carbohydrates, 2% fat)

For a little zing, try adding a tablespoon of miso and a teaspoon of sweetener such as barley malt.

∇ Remember, you can eat the skin and all, so wash it well before you prepare it.

Vegetable Stew

It's probably no surprise to you that beef stew is generally very high in fat (12 grams or 49% fat per cup). As you know, beef in general is very high in fat. An average cut of beef can consist of as much as 75% fat (by calories), and, to make things worse, the fat from the meat melts into the sauce in stew. In contrast, a vegetable stew (ratatouille, for example) has about 5% fat…and, if you like stew to begin with, you won't miss the beef. Here's a stew recipe you'll probably like.

Savory Stew

3 Tbsp.	Water
1 large	Onion, chopped
2 cloves	Garlic, minced
1 piece	Ginger (1"), mashed
1 box	Seitan (wheat gluten), cut in 1" pieces or 1 C mushrooms
1 Tbsp.	Soy sauce
2 large	Carrots, cut in 1" chunks
2 stalks	Celery, cut in 1" chunks
3	Red potatoes, quartered
1 can	Tomatoes, whole packed
3	Bay leaves
2C	Vegetable broth Water, to cover
	Salt, to taste
	Pepper, to taste
2 Tbsp.	Whole wheat flour dissolved in 4 Tbsp. water

Sauté onion and garlic in 3 tablespoons of water in a large pot. Add seitan, ginger, soy sauce, carrots, celery, potatoes, tomatoes, vegetable broth, water to cover, salt, pepper, and bay leaves. Cook until vegetables are tender.   Thicken with whole wheat flour dissolved in 4 tablespoons of water. Serve hot. Zing it with a few drops of Tabasco sauce. Makes 6 to 8 portions. (1 portion = 256.1 calories, 1.2 grams fat, 32% protein, 64% carbohydrates, 4% fat)

Curry Stew

3 Tbsp.	Water
1 lg.	Onion, chopped
2 cloves	Garlic, minced
1 piece	Ginger (1"), mashed
1-2 tsp.	Soy sauce
1 tsp.	Honey
1-3 Tbsp.	Curry powder
2 lg.	Carrots, cut in 1" chunks
2 stalks	Celery, cut in 1" chunks
3	Red potatoes, quartered
3C	Cauliflower florets
½C	Lima beans, frozen
2C	Vegetable broth
	Water, to cover
	Salt, to taste
1 Tbsp.	Corn starch or arrowroot dissolved in 1 tablespoon water

Sauté onion and garlic in 3 tablespoons of water in stainless steel saucepan. Add ginger, soy sauce, honey, curry powder, carrots, celery, potatoes, cauliflower, lima beans, vegetable broth, water to cover, and salt to taste.

Cook for 20 minutes or until carrots become tender. Then thicken with corn starch or arrowroot mixture. Makes 6 portions. (1 portion = 118.5 calories, 0.6 grams fat, 15% protein, 81% carbohydrates, 4% fat)

Nishime (a form of Japanese stew)

This is a traditional Japanese stew-like dish that is low fat and was one of the favorite dishes on both the HawaiiDiet™ Study and the Program.

2strips	Konbu (dried)
4 pieces	Mushrooms (dried)
2	Konyaku,* sliced
3	Aburage*
1C	Turnip
2C	Japanese taro
1C	Bamboo shoots
1C	Carrots
1C	Burdock root
1 tsp.	Peanut oil
1-1/2 C	Vegetable broth
1/4 C	Tamari
1/3 C	Sugar

Soak konbu and mushrooms in water until soft, about 10 minutes.

Wash and scrub Japanese taro thoroughly until clean. Peel and cut into 1-1/2" pieces.

Cut konbu, konyaku, aburage, turnip, bamboo shoots, and carrots into 1-1/2" pieces. Cut burdock root into 1/4"-thick diagonal slices and soak in water until used.

Tie konbu into knots leaving 1" apart. Cut between knots.

In a saucepan, add peanut oil, vegetable broth, mush-rooms, konbu, konyaku, and bamboo shoots. Cover and cook for 10 minutes. Add tamari and sugar; cook for 5 minutes. Add turnip, carrots, and burdock root and cook for 15 minutes. Add taro and cook until taro is fork tender.

Toss in aburage and serve.

Makes 4 portions. Taro must be cooked properly. Do NOT eat raw.

* Konnyaku is a chewy product made from yam flour. Aburage is fried tofu skin, also used for cone sushi. Both are available where Japanese foods are sold.

Monk's Food

This Peace Diet recipe section wouldn't be complete without an example of a recipe for Chinese "monk's food" or "Jai". It is the quintessential dish that represents the ancient belief that vegetarian food helps to nurture the spirit. It has remained in Chinese tradition prominently enough that most Chinese restaurants will serve "Jai" or "Chai" at Chinese New Year because it is supposed to be a dish that helps to cleanse the soul. It is always purely vegan with an assortment of exotic vegetables and other non-animal ingredients. They usually have 10 or more ingredients, some of them quite exotic and difficult to find such as "wood ear" or black fungus, lotus seeds, and lily flowers. If you can find these items, please add them, but this is a recipe with ingredients that are easier to find.

Lo Han Jai (Lo Han means "enlightened person" Jai means vegetarian dish)

6-8 oz Long rice, thin diameter,
5 pieces, Shitake Mushroom, soaked & quartered
1/2 pkg or 6 oz, Flavored or plain firm tofu, cubed
1/2 inch thick piece, Ginger, thinly sliced
2-3 C Won Bok or Chinese Cabbage, cut into thick vertical slices
1/2, Carrot, thinly sliced
½ C, Snow peas, whole or halved
½ C* Canned water chestnuts,
1-2 tsp Tamari soy sauce (or any light to medium colored soy sauce),
2 Tbsp Vegetarian Mushroom Sauce, or 2 tsp Better Than Bouillion Veggie Base,
½ C Water to dilute mushroom sauce or veggie base,
1 Tbsp Cornstarch,
Water to mix in corn starch, 1 C

Maple syrup, 1 t
Sea salt, 2 t or to taste
Chili flakes, a big pinch (optional)
Cooking oil, 2 T

Cut long rice in half and soak in water for ten minutes. Boil in hot water until softened. Drain and set aside. Soak shitake mushroom until pliable and cut each piece into quarters. Squeeze out water. Heat wok or frying pan with 2 t of oil and sautee ginger and mushrooms in medium low heat. Add ½ C of water or more if necessary and cook until mushrooms are tender. Remove from pan.

Fry Tofu cubes in 1 t of oil in medium low heat until golden brown. Remove from pan.

Fry carrots in remaining oil in high heat for 2-3 minutes before adding remaining vegetables. Cook for 3 more minutes. Reduce heat to medium low and add in tofu, sautéed mushrooms and long rice. Combine well and cook for a few more minutes.
Stir in seasoning and pour in cornstarch and water mixture and cook for 2-3 minutes in low heat. Add more water if necessary to ensure perfect consistency. Allow long rice to absorb all or most of the liquid. Remove from wok and serve immediately. Serves 2-3.

Notes: Water chestnuts can be substituted with cooked lotus seeds or roasted peanuts. Cooking oil for frying can be substituted with water or vegetable broth. Provided Courtesy of OriAnn Li, Author, Vegan Paradise, www.oriannli.com

Vegetable Kebobs

Here's an experiment for you. Try taking a piece of meat and chewing it about 100 times. You will for the first time learn the true taste of meat. It tastes like cardboard or worse.

Kebobs taste good because of the sauce, so you don't need the meat. The trick is to get the right sauce. One was so good that one of my patients took vegetable kebobs to a party, used the Dijon marinade and found that even the meat eaters enjoyed them. In fact, they liked the dish so much, they were taking the meat off their kebobs, using my friend's sauce, and enjoying a better tasting kebob.

Simple Vegetable Kebab:

• Try vegetable kebobs with vegetables of your choice such as broccoli, mushrooms, zucchini, onions, cauliflower, bell peppers, or carrots.   Cut them into chunks and place them on skewers. Marinate thoroughly with your favorite marinade sauce.   Then, roast over an open fire or grill.

• Use one of the sauces below. Personally, my favorite is the Dijon Sauce.

(Kebab recipe see at p. 173)

Dijon Mustard Sauce

One of my favorite sauces is what I call "3221" sauce. This is a lip-smacking mustard sauce that can be used to make vegetables absolutely delicious. It's also simple to prepare.

It's called "3221" because you use:

3 Tbsp.	Dijon mustard
2 Tbsp.	Soy sauce
2 Tbsp.	Lemon juice or balsamic vinegar
1 clove	Garlic, crushed

Mix them all togjether, and you have a delicious dipping sauce that is out of this world. It's incredibly easy. Try it and see. Makes 3 portions. (1 portion = 25.6 calories, 0.6 grams fat, 26% protein, 52% carbohydrates, 22% fat)

Asian Sauce

Oriental sauce is delicious on vegetables.

You can make a variety of these sauces from scratch, or buy them bottled. Also, for your convenience, you can use a vegetarian oyster sauce, a miso sauce, or a ginger sauce. Ginger is a superb condiment and can be used as an ingredient in any number of different sauces. Ginger has a little bit of zip, similar to horseradish or chili sauce.

Oriental Ginger Sauce

1C	Water
4 Tbsp.	Low-sodium soy sauce
1 Tbsp.	Arrowroot or corn starch
1 Tbsp.	Ginger, grated

Mix arrowroot or corn starch in ¼ cup of cool water. Add to a saucepan with the water, soy sauce, and ginger. Heat at medium until thickened and stir.

Serve with steamed vegetables. Makes 10 portions. (1 portion = 6.9 calories, 0.0 grams fat, 21% protein, 78% carbohydrates, 1% fat)

Plum Sauce (Hoi Sin Sauce)

Oriental plum sauce is a delicious treat
that can be used for dishes such as "Mu-shu" vegetable. One
variation of plum sauce is known as "Hoisin." You can buy this
bottled, and use it as is. You'll find it in Oriental or health food
stores.

Miso-Based Sauce

Miso-based sauces are also savory on
vegetables. All you have to do is dilute some miso with a little bit
of flour, water and other spices, then use this as a delicious
dipping sauce for raw or steamed vegetables. You can also use
this sauce as a variation when you're making a stir-fry.

Ginger Miso Sauce

4 Tbsp.	Sweet white miso
1 Tbsp.	Fresh ginger juice
1 Tbsp.	Ginger, grated
1 clove	Garlic (large), minced
1	Juice of one lemon
½ tsp.	Corn starch (for thicker sauce)
1C	Water

Blend ingredients until well mixed, then heat gently. Add corn starch for a thicker sauce. Serve over vegetables, use as dipping sauce, or use as base in stir-frys. Keeps well. Makes 8 portions. (1 portion = 22.7 calories, 0.6 grams fat, 19% protein, 59% carbohydrates, 21% fat)

Barbecue Sauce

Barbecue sauces are great for dressing up vegetables. They also make good sauces for sandwich fillings and protein-based foods such as the meat substitutes.

You can make your own sauce, or barbecue sauce can be bought in the store. Most of these sauces are low in fat. Nevertheless, make sure that you read the bottle or you might be surprised.

The brands of bottled barbecue sauces I recommend include the following: Robbie's Barbecue Sauce®, Hickory Flavor; Bull's Eye Original Barbecue Sauce®; and Hunt's All Natural Thick & Rich Barbecue Sauce®, to name a few.

BBQ Sauce

½C	Water
1 tsp.	Soy sauce
1 large	Onion, minced
3 cloves	Garlic, minced
1 can	Tomato sauce (8 oz.)
1C	Tomato ketchup
1C	Water
1 Tbsp.	Honey
1 tsp.	Chili powder
2 Tbsp.	Cider vinegar
1 tsp.	Dry mustard
2 Tbsp.	Tamari
½ Tbsp.	Corn starch, whole wheat flour, dissolved in 2 tablespoons water

In a large pan, heat water and soy sauce.

Add chopped onion and the garlic. Cook until the onion is soft. Add other ingredients and cook over medium heat for 10 minutes. Stir often.

To thicken, add corn starch, whole wheat flour, or kuzu, dissolved in water. Makes 36 portions. (1 portion = 22.8 calories, 0.1 grams fat, 10% protein, 85% carbohydrates, 5% fat)

Kebob Salad

2C	Firm tofu cubes or Tofu Nuggets
1 large	Red bell pepper
1 large	Green bell pepper
1 large	Yellow bell pepper
16	Cherry tomatoes
16 Fresh	pineapple chunks
16	Button mushrooms 1 med.
	Zucchini
2-3 Tbsp.	Any of this cookbook's dressings

Shredded lettuce for bed

Wash all vegetables well. Cut all the bell peppers into small, equal-sized chunks.

Skewer the tofu cubes or nuggets, peppers, tomatoes, pineapple chunks, and mushrooms onto wooden kebab sticks, alternating the colors and textures, starting and ending with a cherry tomato.

Arrange on shredded bed of lettuce on platter, drizzle favorite dressing over bed of kebabs, to taste. *Makes 4 portions. (1 portion = 296.5 calories, 12.3 grams fat, 30% protein, 37% carbohydrates, 33% fat - dressing not included)*

Salads and Dressings

Salads are super high on the SMI scale. They're one of the easiest and tastiest ways to eat your high-SMI foods. If you enjoy a salad as a main course for lunch or dinner, you can get your daily requirement of vegetables all at once. Since salads often consist of all raw foods, they have a natural balance of fiber, nutrients, and water that your body needs. While cooking food can deplete vitamins, destroy enzymes that help digestion, and even damage fats and proteins, this does not happen to salads, which are raw food in its natural state. They have no processed foods or additives to worry about.

However, there is one key problem. Most people ruin their salads before they take their first bite by dousing them with oily, high-fat salad dressings. Oily salad dressings are the lowest in SMI of all foods. They'll instantly ruin the weight-loss value of a salad. The trick is to use salad dressings that are medium to high in SMI and contain little or no oil. This is not hard to do with a little work, as you will see in the section below on salad dressings.

Besides using medium to high SMI dressings, you can choose to try different types of salads that don't rely quite so heavily on the dressing. There are many of varieties: corn salads, beet salads, three-bean salads and others that will delight your taste buds without tempting you to resort to high-fat dressings. Some cold noodle dishes also adapt well to salad recipes. Or you can modify the following to create your own.

Salad Dressings

Papaya Seed Dressing*

1	Papaya (ripe) Seeds of 1/3 papaya
1 Tbsp.	Dijon mustard
2-3 Tbsp.	Balsamic or red wine vinegar
1 Tbsp.	Soy sauce

Slice one ripe papaya in half, discarding all but 1/3 of the seeds. Scoop out flesh of the papaya and put into blender. Add in the rest of the ingredients and blend on high until smooth.

Makes 10 portions (about 1+ cups).   (1 portion = 8 calories, 0.0 gram fat, 12% protein, 82% carbohydrates, 5% fat)

* From Dick Allgire in Dr. Shintani's Eat More, Weigh Less® Cookbook, page 198

Pineapple Miso Dressing

2C	Pineapple juice, unsweetened
1/2 C	White miso
	1 medium Maui onion (mild, sweet . onion), chopped
2 Tbsp.	Ginger, peeled and minced
1/4 C	Soy sauce, or to taste
1 Tbsp.	Balsamic vinegar (for fragrance) . White pepper, to taste

Blend all the above ingredients together.
Variation:

Substitute pineapple juice with fresh papaya,
mandarin oranges, or canned fruit juice.
*Makes 24 portions (about 4 cups).   (1   portion   =   28   calories,   0.4
grams fat, 15% protein, 73% carbohydrates, 12% fat)*

Mark Ellman's Tomato Miso Vinaigrette

Tomato miso vinaigrette was probably the favorite dressing on the Hawaii Health Program. You will enjoy the Pacific Rim tastes of this dressing, too.

2 Tbsp.	Onion, chopped
1C	White wine
1/2 tsp.	Garlic, chopped
2	sprigs Tarragon (fresh)
1C	Rice vinegar
1C	Tomato purée
8 Tbsp.	Red miso
1 tsp.	Sesame seed oil
3 tsp.	Extra virgin olive oil

Sauté onion and garlic in wine. Reduce to a glacé.

Add vinegar and reduce by one-half. Add tomato and tarragon. Reduce by one-half and add red miso. Boil once. Emulsify in blender with olive oil and fresh tarragon, with a touch of sesame seed oil. Add water if too thick.

Makes 24 portions.   (1 portion = 31 calories, 1.1 grams fat, 14% protein, 49% carbohydrates, 37% fat)

Thousand Island Dressing

No, this is not the usual high fat version! This one is so good that many people believe that it is "illegal," but when you see that the fat content is less than one gram per serving you'll want to use it more often.

1/4 C	Water
1/8 tsp.	Salt
1/8 tsp.	Pepper
1 tsp.	Seasoned salt
2 Tbsp.	Tomato ketchup
1C	Tofu (soft), crumbled
4 sprigs	Parsley (fresh) (optional)
1 Tbsp.	Cucumber, chopped fine
1 Tbsp.	Celery chopped fine or pickle relish

Whiz all ingredients, except cucumber, celery, or pickle relish, in blender. Add cucumber, celery, or pickle relish. Chill and serve.

Makes 12 portions (about 1-1/2 cups). (1 portion = 18 calories, 0.8 gram fat, 34% protein, 26% carbohydrates, 40% fat)

Tangy Dijon Dressing

Even the most finicky eaters will come back for more of this delicious salad dressing.

1 Tbsp.	Extra Virgin Olive oil
2/3 C	Water
4-1/2 Tbsp.	White wine vinegar
2-3 cloves	Garlic, minced
4 tsp.	Dijon mustard
1/4 tsp.	Thyme
1/2 tsp.	Salt
1/4 tsp.	Pepper
2 tsp.	Sugar or honey

Mix all ingredients, store in a container, and refrigerate.

Makes 8 portions.   (1 portion = 24 calories, 1.8 grams fat, 2% protein, 31% carbohydrates, 67% fat)

Oriental Vinaigrette Dressing

For an Oriental flair, add this dressing to vegetables such as won bok, water chestnuts, bean sprouts, or jicama.

4 Tbsp.	Vinegar
4 Tbsp.	Soy sauce
2 Tbsp.	Water
1 tsp.	Sesame oil
1 tsp.	Extra Virgin Olive oil
1 Tbsp.	Mustard
2 Tbsp.	Sugar or honey

Combine all ingredients and refrigerate.

Makes 6 portions.   (1 portion = 39 calories, 1.6 grams fat, 11% protein, 55% carbohydrates, 34% fat)

Balsamic Vinaigrette

The secret ingredient to this dressing is the balsamic vinegar. It is great as a dressing ingredient because like all vinegars it has no fat or cholesterol, and it has a savory, tangy taste without the sour smell of some vinegars.

1/3 C	Balsamic vinegar
1/4 C	Apple cider vinegar
1/4 C	Water
1 Tbsp.	Dijon mustard
1 Tbsp.	Garlic (fresh), minced
1 Tbsp.	Olive oil
1 Tbsp.	Parsley (fresh), minced
2 Tbsp.	Apple juice concentrate

Place ingredients in a small bowl. Whisk together and let sit for at least 15 minutes to allow flavors to meld. Toss with your favorite green salad or pasta salad.

Makes 8 portions.   (1 portion = 25 calories, 1.7 grams fat, 1% protein, 43% carbohydrates, 56% fat)

Chinese Lettuce Wraps

Any type of green lettuce leaves---cut/break into nice shapes for wrapping (green, red, butter, small romaine leaves, or manoa lettuce are the best to use).

Filling

1 cup	round onions chopped small but not minced
2 cloves	minced or pressed garlic
2 tspn	grated ginger
2 Tbsp	soy sauce

(For more flavor, season with mushroom powder as desired if adding more ingredients.)

2 Tblspn	pure maple syrup
I Tbsp	mirin (sweet japanese rice wine vinegar)
1 small can	water chestnuts, drained and finely chopped
1 large can	bamboo strips, drained, rinsed, and chopped
1 cup	chopped mushrooms
1 Tblspn	ground sesame seeds (optional)
	Chopped cilantro (optional)

Thinly sliced green onions (optional)
Minced celery (optional)
(Don't make mixture too salty since you will be adding soy dressing w/wrap.)
1 cup "ground round" style seitan (wheat gluten)
(more seitan can be added for larger serving)
Note: If seitan is not available, use Mrs. Chen's baked tofu or any other brand of baked tofu (chop/add quantity desired). Meatless Ground (NonGMO Soy from COSTCO) can also be used (comes in green box).

Start off by sauteing onions, ginger, and garlic in a few teaspoons of sesame oil. If too dry, add a few teaspoons of water (a little at a time instead of using too much oil). Add chopped mushrooms and keep stirring to cook. Then add chestnuts and bamboo shoots. Keep sautéing and then add soy sauce, maple syrup, and mirin, stirring completely (adjust your heat). When everything looks cooked, add the seitan or baked tofu last. Sprinkle sesame seeds---keep stirring until done.   Place in large serving bowl. Sprinkle thinly sliced green onions and then more sesame seeds on top before serving with lettuce.

Soy dressing (to drizzle on to filling to be wrapped in lettuce):

Mix together 2 Tblspn brown rice vinegar, 3 Tblspn maple syrup, 1 Tblspn mirin,3/4 Cup soy sauce, 2 tspn minced/or pressed garlic.
Add to taste, minced/mashed green chili peppers (about a teaspoon).

Note: Hawaiian green chili peppers seem to have the best flavor when adding to soy sauce dressings. Buy a small handful (from Chinatown okay) and freeze it for future use (since you probably will use only one chili pepper at a time).

High Calcium Vegetables

Many people have been raised on dairy, so they automatically see that as the natural source for calcium. They don't realize that vegetables are actually the best source of calcium. Think for a minute. After all, where do cows get calcium? They don't eat dairy. They eat greens. And if you are concerned about osteoporosis, remember that the countries that consume the most dairy have the most osteoporosis in their population. So where do we get calcium?

Fortunately, nature provides plenty of calcium in dark leafy greens and sea vegetables. Steam or par-boil them and if you wish, flavor them with one of the sauces described in this book for kebabs. Here are some examples that you can use as high calcium side dishes.

- Broccoli is one of the best sources of calcium. One-half cup daily exceeds the recommended daily allowance (RDA) of both vitamin C and E.
- Kale contains more calcium than milk, ounce for ounce. Its calcium is more absorbable by the body than milk. Its calcium protects against osteoporosis, arthritis, and bone loss.
- Collard greens include not only calcium but also the key ingredients of iron, magnesium, potassium, sodium, zinc, copper, manganese, vitamin C, B, E, and several phytochemicals.
- Watercress is an excellent source of calcium and antioxidants for fighting cancer, but also treats anemia, calcium deficiencies, liver and pancreatic problems, thyroid problems, and arthritis.

- Beet or turnip greens provide calcium, minerals, and carotenes. They provide vitamins and phytochemicals.
- Bok choy is an excellent source of highly absorbable calcium as well as beta-carotene to battle heart disease and cancer.
- Mustard cabbage (napa cabbage) also contains highly absorbable calcium and iron. It protects against cancer and heart disease and strengthens the immune system.

Other good sources of calcium are wakame and kelp (sea vegetables, see below).   Don't forget that there is also a fair amount of calcium in beans as well.

Taking a calcium supplement with magnesium and vitamin D is another option if you are sure you won't be eating greens.

Zesty Broccoli

1 bunch	broccoli
1	lemon or lemon juice
2 tsp	garlic powder
	soy sauce to taste

Wash the broccoli and peel off the fibrous part of the stem. Then cut into bite-sized flowerets. Steam or par-boil until barely fork-tender and still bright green. Drain the water and then, squeeze lemon juice onto each floweret. Then sprinkle the garlic powder and a little soy sauce or Bragg's liquid aminos to taste. (Hint: if you have a Bragg's liquid amino spray bottle, it is easier to distribute the soy sauce or liquid aminos evenly).

Sea Vegetables

Sea vegetables come in many varieties. We associate them with Japan and China, but really they are collected from all over the world. It is marine algae which grows in shallow waters on ocean shores.

These exotic vegetables supply our greatest source of minerals and trace elements. They contain alginic acid which has the ability to detoxify the body by binding with any heavy metals and causing them to be released from our bodies. Sea vegetables are also high in protein and fiber, with significant amounts of calcium, iron, potassium, phosphorus, magnesium, zinc, iodine, and vitamins A, C, E, K, and B-complex.

Probably the easiest way to use seaweed is to add it to soup. You can add wakame to any soup you can think of and it will add an excellent source of minerals and flavor. Soup recipes are in the section following these seaweed side dishes.

Wakame with Onions

1 oz.	Wakame (dry weight)
1-2	Onions, medium- sized
.	Water, as needed
1 Tbsp.	Low-sodium soy sauce

Rinse, and soak the wakame in water until tender, then slice into roughly 1" pieces. Peel and slice onions vertically into crescents. Place onions in a pot, then cover with wakame. Add water to nearly cover the wakame.

Bring the mixture to a boil, and reduce the heat to low. Simmer for about 15 minutes. Season with low-sodium soy sauce to taste, and cook for 10 minutes longer. Makes 4 to 6 portions. (1 portion = 16.5 calories, 0.1 grams fat, 16% protein, 79% carbohydrates, 4% fat)

Hijiki With Carrots (or other vegetables)

Hijiki is commonly used in japanese-style "shojin ryori" or food for spiritual development. It is a delicious string-like or thread-like sea vegetable that is very high in calcium, iodine and iron (as are virtually all sea vegetables). The trick to making hijiki is to cook it long enough to evaporate the strong ocean aroma that comes out initially, so don't let the initial fragrance prevent you from using it. It is delicious with other vegetables and is loaded with minerals.

1 oz.	Hijiki (dry weight)
½ tsp.	Sesame oil
2	Carrots or other vegetables such as onions, burdock root, lotus root, corn, or tofu
	Water, as needed
	Low-sodium soy sauce to taste

Wakame with Mixed Vegetables

Wakame

Wakame with mixed vegetables is another high calcium dish primarily because of the seaweed (wakame).

2-1/2 oz.	Wakame, dried
5C	Daikon, sliced
5C	Carrots, diced
5C	Cauliflower, cut
5C	Turnips, sliced
8 Tbsp.	Soy sauce (low sodium)
	Water, Green Onions (garnish)

Rinse and soak wakame. Slice into large pieces.

Put other vegetables in a large soup pot and half cover with water. Bring to a boil, cover, and reduce heat to low, simmering until the vegetables are almost cooked. Add wakame and low-sodium soy sauce to taste until the vegetables are cooked.

Serve one cup in a bowl and garnish with green onions.

Makes 20 portions. (1 portion = 47 calories, 0.3 grams fat, 17% protein, 78% carbohydrates, 5% fat)

Hijiki

2 to 3 Tbsp. Sweetener such as barley
dash   malt (optional)

Wash and rinse the hijiki in a strainer or colander. After washing, be sure to place in a separate bowl to drain to eliminate any sand that may be present. Then soak hijiki for about 10 minutes. While soaking, slice the carrots into julienned sticks. Lightly oil a frying pan, and heat it. Add the carrots and a little water and sauté for 2 to 3 minutes. Place the hijiki on top of the carrots and add water to cover the mixture.

Bring to a boil, turn the heat to low, then add a small amount of low-sodium soy sauce. Cover and simmer for about 40 minutes (depending on the vegetable). Add soy sauce to taste. Simmer for another 15 minutes, or until the liquid is almost gone. Makes 4 to 6 portions.

(1 portion = 36.3 calories, 0.6 grams fat, 14% protein, 72% carbohydrates, 14% fat)

Soups

Soups have always been the way to get a lot of ingredients – and a lot of nutrition – into one pot at one time, tasty and easy to make. Plant-based soups are no exception; in fact, it's even truer for them. A bowl of soup, a slice of whole-grain bread, and a piece of fruit for dessert – Voila! A feast.

One of the best tasting soups is almost an "instant" soup. Basmati may be the King of Rice, but miso is the Queen of Soups. In fact, the two can make a perfect match in a variety of menus.

Miso is made from fermented soybean paste. It is a traditional Japanese soup base that has served Asian chefs well for centuries. Deliciously robust, highly nutritious, this soup stock is simple and easy to prepare. Today, miso can be found in supermarkets and in health food stores. You can also find various types of miso in Oriental food stores. More and more people are appreciating and seeking out Asian foods.

ALMOST INSTANT: To make basic miso soup (Zip Miso Soup), boil water and just before serving dissolve some miso in it, as described below. Make sure it is blended smoothly to get the lumps out. Garnish it with some chopped green onions or seaweed, and it's ready to serve. For one variety of miso soup, simply prepare some of your favorite vegetables in water. Just before you serve them, dissolve the miso into the hot water, and you've created a delicious miso-based soup. Miso is very high in protein, so it is a great substitute for any animal product-based soup. It is also quite high in sodium. However, this can be controlled by the amount of miso you use per cup of hot water.

For Some Variety, Try...

Miso cam be used to season all types of soups, and it can flavor and add nutrition to sauces, gravies, salad dressings, dips, casseroles, and vegetables...it can even be used as a marinade.

Try miso soup for breakfast or with dinner.

Try the following miso recipes for a variation that will satisfy your appetite for something special.

Breakfast Miso Soup

2½ C	Water
1	Wakame seaweed (3" strip)
1/8 C	Firm tofu, chopped to ½" chunks
1	Green onion, with stems, chopped fine
1 Tbsp.	Barley miso

Bring water to a boil, add wakame and one-half of green onion, simmer 5 minutes.

Turn off heat, add miso to taste by diluting 1 to 2 tablespoons of miso in a ladle full of the soup water, mashing and smoothing out the miso and adding it back to the pot.

Pour into a large bowl, over small chunks of tofu. Garnish with chopped green onions, serve steaming hot.

Makes 4 to 6 portions. (1 portion = 18.1 calories, 0.8 grams fat, 30% protein, 34% carbohydrates, 35% fat)

Portuguese Bean Soup*

This version of a traditional Portuguese favorite is low-fat, no cholesterol, and full-flavored despite the absence of meat. The flavor is retained because of the use of spices.

6 cloves	Garlic, crushed
1-1/2	Round onions, chopped
2 stalks	Celery, chopped
4	Carrots, diced
1 can	Vegetable broth (14-1/2 oz.)
2 cans	Whole tomatoes plus juice (large), cut in chunks
3	Potatoes, cubed
3C	Beans, cooked
1/2 head	Cabbage, chopped
1C	Macaroni, cooked

Sauté garlic and onions in 2 cups water until transparent. Add celery and carrots. Continue cooking 5 minutes. Add tomatoes and vegetable broth. Add 2 cups more water to mixture. Cook 15 minutes, then add remainder of ingredients, except beans and macaroni. Continue to cook 30 minutes on warm setting, after bringing to a boil. Add beans and simmer on warm for 30 minutes, until done to taste. Add cooked macaroni a few minutes before serving.

Makes 8 portions. (1 portion = 231 calories, 1.0 gram fat, 20% protein, 76% carbohydrates, 4% fat)

Presto Minestrone

4 cloves	Garlic, minced
1	Onion, minced
1	Carrot, cut into 1/2" slices
1	stalk Celery
1	Potato, cut into 1/2" pieces
1C	Peas, frozen
2 cans	Italian stewed tomatoes
2 cans	Water
1/2 C	Whole wheat elbow macaroni

Sauté garlic and onions in 2 to 4 tablespoons of water. Add remaining ingredients and simmer for 30 minutes. Add macaroni and boil until macaroni is tender, about 10 minutes.

Makes 8 portions (8 cups). (1 portion = 97 calories, 0.4 gram fat, 14% protein, 82% carbohydrates, 4% fat)

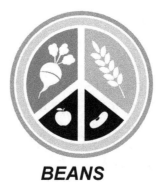

BEANS

Beans are delicious, hearty and filling and a great source of protein and iron. They can be caloric dense, but they can be excellent weight loss dishes when prepared properly. Moderate to high on the SMI, they make delicious dips and spreads that are very low in fat (as long as you don't add any fats).

From a health standpoint, beans are not only fat free but research associates them with lower rates of heart disease and some cancers. Beans provide significant amounts of folate, manganese, magnesium, copper, iron, and potassium – nutrients we don't always get enough of.

Beans come in a variety of shapes, colors, and sizes, which add interest to cooking and eating. Dried beans are the least expensive, but take longer to prepare. They last for a year or more in an airtight container.

If you don't have time to cook, pick up a can at the supermarket or the health food store. Simply drain and use these beans as if they were cooked beans.

Chunky 2-Bean Chili

Although chili is a favorite bean dish in America, there are many ways to make it.   At one of our cooking sessions, this was the favorite recipe.

1/3 C	Vegetable broth
1C	TVP (textured vegetable protein)
3 cloves	Garlic, chopped
1/2	Onion, chopped
1 stalk	Celery, chopped
1	Green pepper, chopped
1 sprig	Cilantro (Chinese parsley), chopped
1-2 Tbsp.	Chili powder
1/2 tsp.	Red pepper flakes
1 tsp.	Cumin
	Black pepper, to taste
2C	Kidney beans, (cooked or canned), drained or rinsed
2C	Black beans, (cooked or canned), drained or rinsed
2	Bay leaves
1C	Tomato sauce
1/2 C	Tomato paste
1/2 C	Water
1 tsp.	Lime juice

Soak the TVP in the broth. Sauté garlic, onion, celery, green pepper, and cilantro in some vegetable broth. Add the soaked TVP and remaining ingredients to the mixture and simmer. Adjust seasonings to taste. Remove bay leaves before serving. Make the day before for better flavor. Makes 8 portions. (1 portion = 186 calories, 0.9 gram fat, 39% protein, 57% carbohydrates, 4% fat)

Tofu Nuggets

1 blk.	Firm tofu, cut in ¾" cubes
1/3 C	Nutritional yeast
1 tsp.	Spike® seasoning or vegetarian chicken broth powder
½ tsp.	Black pepper
1½ Tbsp.	Soy sauce or tamari
¼ tsp.	Olive or sesame oil (or cooking spray)

Slice or break tofu into approximately ¾" cubes. Coat nonstick pan with oil or cooking spray and heat at medium-high. Add tofu cubes and brown. Turn heat to low and drizzle soy sauce on each piece of tofu. Add yeast, Spike®, and pepper and toss, coating the pieces of tofu evenly. Cook until golden brown. Makes 2 to 4 portions. (1 portion = 118.2 calories, 3.6 grams fat, 45% protein, 29% carbohydrates, 26% fat)

Srambled Tofu*

Scrambled Tofu is a delicious substitute for scrambled eggs. The best reason to replace eggs for breakfast is the 430 mg. of cholesterol found in two eggs (more than the amount of cholesterol in an 8-ounce steak). Tofu, of course, as in any plant-based product,
has no cholesterol.

1 block	Tofu, firm
1/4 C	Onions, minced
2 tsp.	Vegetarian "chicken-flavored" seasoning
1/2 tsp.	Turmeric
1/4 tsp.	Sea salt
1/4 tsp.	Onion powder
1/4 tsp.	Garlic powder
	Canola oil cooking spray

Lightly spray a large non-stick skillet with canola oil cooking spray. Sauté onions, adding a slight amount of water if they start to stick. As the onions cook, add sea- sonings and mix.

Break up tofu into scrambled-egg consistency and add to the mixture. Cook until the mixture is thoroughly heated and resembles scrambled eggs.

Serve with whole grain toast or pancakes.
*Makes 5 portions. (1 portion = 95 calories, 4.2 grams
fat, 38% protein, 24% carbohydrates, 38% fat)*
* From Dr. Shintani's Eat More, Weigh Less® Cookbook

Barbecue Baked Beans

1C	Onion, diced
3	cans Beans (14-16 oz. kidney, black, navy, pinto, great northern, lima)
2 Tbsp.	Blackstrap molasses
2 Tbsp.	Apple cider vinegar
1 Tbsp.	Dry mustard
½ tsp.	Garlic powder
½C	Tomato ketchup
	Canola oil cooking spray

Heat oven to 350o F. While heating, sauté onion in an oil-sprayed nonstick pan. Pour off half the liquid from each bean can. Mix beans and remaining ingredients in large bowl and add onion. Mix thoroughly. Put into a 2-quart casserole and bake, uncovered, for 1½ hours, stirring after 1 hour. Makes 4 to 6 portions. (1 portion = 279.1 calories, 1.6 grams fat, 18% protein, 77% carbohydrates, 5% fat)

Maui Tacos' Black Bean Burrito

Rice and beans, the daily fare of many peoples around the world including Latin Americans, do make a healthy combination. Add some potatoes and enjoy this hearty burrito recipe contributed by Chef Mark Ellman of Avalon and Maui Tacos restaurants. If you want this made for you, go to one of the Maui Tacos locations in Napili, Lahaina, Kihei, Kahului, Hilo, and Honolulu.

12 oz.	Rice, cooked or Spanish rice
5 small	Potatoes
1/2	Onion, chopped
1 Tbsp.	Garlic (granulated)
1 tsp.	Salt
1 can	Black beans (16 oz.), or cooked
5	Tortillas (12")
8 oz.	Lettuce, shredded
7 oz.	Salsa or Maui Tacos' Pineapple Tomatillo Salsa
4 oz.	Maui Tacos' Guacamole

Wash and peel potatoes. Place in saucepan and water to cover. Add salt. Boil potatoes for 35 to 40 min-utes. Drain water and cube into 1/2" cubes and set aside. Water-sauté onion and granulated garlic until trans- lucent. Add black beans, potatoes, and rice. Gently mix together until combined. Lay out tortillas on a flat surface. Layer the filling in the following order: black bean-potato-rice mixture, lettuce, salsa, and guacamole. Fold tortilla over layers, envelope fashion. *Makes 5 portions. (1 portion with guacamole = 440 calories, 4.9 grams fat, 13% protein, 77% carbohydrates, 10% fat) (1 portion without guacamole = 416 calories, 2.7 grams fat, 13% protein, 81% carbohydrates, 6% fat)*

Maui Tacos' Black Beans

1 lb.   Black beans, triple washed
         Water, to cover
1/4   Onion, chopped
1 tsp.   Salt
1 Tbsp. Garlic (granulated)

Wash beans thoroughly.
In a large pot, add the beans, onions, salt, garlic,
and enough water to cover beans while cooking. Bring to a boil,
then turn heat to low. Cook for 4 hours or until beans are tender.
Remove from heat. Cool. Leave black beans whole.
Makes 5 portions. (1 portion   = 125 calories, 0.5 gram
fat, 25% protein, 71% carbohydrates, 4% fat)

Simple Hummus

1C	Garbanzo beans, cooked
2-3 Tbsp.	Lemon juice
1 Tbsp.	Onion, minced
1 clove	Garlic, crushed
1 tsp.	Cumin
1 tsp	Sesame seeds, freshly ground
	Low-sodium soy sauce or salt, to taste
	Pepper to taste
	Water

Cook the dry garbanzo beans per package directions. (Also, see bean cooking chart on page 308.) You may use precooked canned beans instead, if you wish. Mash beans and mix ingredients together with enough water to keep a thick moist dip consistency. Makes 8 portions.

(1 portion = 93.5 calories, 1.3 grams fat, 22% protein,
67% carbohydrates, 12% fat)

Mock Tuna

(made w/garbanzo beans)

1   15-oz. can organic garbanzo beans (drained)

Mash garbanzos (fork or potato masher will do if only making a small amount). You may still want to use a food processor to speed up your mashing. Mix following ingredients with beans while mashing:

1/4 tsp   salt
2 tsp   lemon juice
1/4 tsp   pepper
1 tsp   soy sauce
1/2 tsp   Kelp powder
1/2 tsp   Spike Seasoning
(Kelp powder can be purchased at Down to Earth spice jar counter)

After mashing, then add following ingredients and mix well. (Do not food-process beans with these ingredients---just mix it in.)

1/4 Cup   Minced celery
1 Tblspn   Minced round onions or green onions (sliced ft
2 Tblspn   Nutritional yeast
1/2Cup   Fat Free Nayonaise   (or other Fat Free vegan
               mayo)
Use in sandwiches, salads, or as a dip.

Cooking Chart for Beans

1 Cup of Beans	Regular Pot		Pressure Cooker	
	Cups Water	Time	Cups Water	Time
Lentils	3	30-60 min.	to cover	10-20 min.
Split Peas	2-3	30-60 min.	½" over	10 min.
Black Beans	4	1.5-2 hrs.	¾" over	10-20 min.
Kidney Beans	3	1.5-2 hrs.	½" over	15-20 min.
Navy Beans	2	1.5-2 hrs.	½" over	10-20 min.
Pinto Beans	3	2-2.5 hrs.	½" over	10-15 min.
Chickpeas (garbanzos)	2	2.5-3 hrs.	½" over	15-25 min.
Azuki Beans	3	2-2.5 hrs.	½" over	15-20 min.
Soy Beans	3-4	3-4 hrs.	¾" over	30 min.

Portuguese Bean Soup

This version of a traditional Portuguese favorite is low-fat, no cholesterol, and full-flavored despite the absence of meat. The flavor is retained because of the use of spices.

6 cloves	Garlic, crushed
1-1/2	Round onions, chopped
2 stalks	Celery, chopped
4	Carrots, diced
1 can	Vegetable broth (14-1/2 oz.)
2 cans	Whole tomatoes plus juice (large), cut in chunks
3	Potatoes, cubed
3C	Beans, cooked
1/2 head	Cabbage, chopped
1C	Macaroni, cooked

Sauté garlic and onions in 2 cups water until transparent. Add celery and carrots. Continue cooking 5 minutes. Add tomatoes and vegetable broth. Add 2 cups more water to mixture. Cook 15 minutes, then add remainder of ingredients, except beans and macaroni. Continue to cook 30 minutes on warm setting, after bringing to a boil. Add beans and simmer on warm for 30 minutes, until done to taste. Add cooked macaroni a few minutes before serving.

Makes 8 portions.   (1 portion = 231 calories, 1.0 gram fat, 20% protein, 76% carbohydrates, 4% fat)

Potato and Corn Chowder

Probably the best liked soup on the Hawaii Health Program.

2 tsp.	Dry cooking sherry
1-1/4 C	Sweet yellow onion, finely chopped
2 cloves	Garlic, crushed
2C	Red potatoes, cubed
1 can	Vegetable stock (14-1/4 oz.)
1C	Soy milk
1C	Corn kernels (fresh or frozen)
1	Bay leaf
1/4 tsp.	Paprika
1/4 tsp.	Thyme
1 tsp.	Basil
	Salt, to taste
	Pepper, to taste
	Olive oil cooking spray

Add wine to a large oil-sprayed skillet and heat. Add onions and garlic and sauté for 5 minutes, stirring frequently to prevent browning. Add water as needed.

Add potatoes, bay leaf, herbs, and stock to sautéed onions and garlic. Cover pan, bring to a boil, and cook over medium heat for 10 to 15 minutes.

When the potatoes are tender, add the corn and milk. Simmer until the corn is tender, about 3 minutes. Discard the bay leaf.

Use your hand blender to partially purée the mixture, or remove a cup of soup and purée in blender or food processor, then return it to the pot. This will give your soup a creamy texture. Season with salt and/or pepper to taste.

Makes 6 to 8 portions. (1 portion = 117 calories, 1.3 grams fat, 18% protein, 70% carbohydrates, 10% fat)

This and other cream soups are a snap to make if you have a hand blender. With this, you can partially blend the soup right in the pot. Just wait until it's almost done then do your blending, leaving enough chunky ingredients to give the soup texture. Watch out for spattering though, if it's really hot.

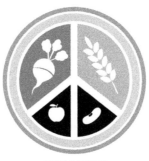

FRUITS

Most fruits are high on the SMI scale and as a result will not contribute to weight gain. They also contain a wealth of vitamins and phytonutrients such as beta- carotene and vitamin C. But fruit has relatively high sugar content. Fructose, the natural sugar in fruit, can be absorbed very quickly. It's not as bad as white sugar, but it's still not good for you in large amounts. As with processed sugars, it tends to cause a rise in triglycerides (storage fats) in our blood. High triglycerides are a co-risk factor with cholesterol for heart disease.

Have a piece of raw fruit, such as an orange, apple, blueberries or other treat, either as a snack or for breakfast. It's portable, so very convenient as a snack or a breakfast on the go. Use fruits as a dessert to satisfy your sweet tooth, but don't eat too much fruit. Two to four servings is fine for most people. Fruit – easy access and easier preparation. Yet, research shows that, even though people who eat fruit regularly have reduced rates of all cancers, heart disease, and other illnesses, half of all Americans don't eat fruit at all. Moderation is the key here.

Eating the whole fruit is better than drinking fruit juice or consuming fruit smoothies. Liquefying fruit or any food tends to raise the glycemic index of the food. In other words, processing the food tends to increase its rate of absorption and raises blood sugar levels and insulin requirement. Some people find that fruits are easier to digest if they are cooked. Others do better with raw fruit. Some people go on "fruit fasts" as an effective way to lose weight. I don't recommend this approach. It would cause weight loss, because fruits are high on the SMI. But I believe a more balanced diet is important for good health. If possible, try to eat fruit in season, and from your own locality.

Whole Fruit

A's Baked Apples

8 medium Apples
1C Apple juice
1 Tbsp. Cinnamon, ground
1/2 tsp. Nutmeg, ground
16 Apricots (dried)

Core apple and slice a small hole in top of apple with a vegetable peeler. Core out seeds, leaving the apple whole. Place apples in a baking dish. Add apple juice, cinnamon, ground nutmeg, and apricots to the baking dish. Spoon some of this liquid into the center of each apple. Cover with tinfoil and bake at 350o F. for 10 minutes. Remove dish from oven, uncover, and pour more liquid into the center of each apple. Cover again and cook for 20 minutes more. Remove dish again from oven, uncover, and add liquid to the center of apples. Cook uncovered for 5 minutes. Apples should be soft, but not mushy. Remove apples and put on platter or individual dishes. Remove apricots from sauce. Chop apricots and add to the center of the apples. Cook sauce until reduced to 1/2 cup. Pour reduced sauce over apples. If you wish, you may drizzle 1/2 teaspoon of honey over each apple. Sprinkle each apple with cinnamon and nutmeg or, as an option, with raisins. Serve warm or cold.

Makes 8 portions. (1 portion = 125 calories, 0.7 gram fat, 2% protein, 94% carbohydrates, 4% fat)

Quick Apple Pie

½C	Grape Nuts® cereal
4C	Delicious apples (large)
2 tsp.	Cinnamon
2 tsp.	Corn starch
2 tsp.	Lemon juice
1/3 C	Frozen apple juice concentrate, thawed
½ tsp.	Ground coriander
¼C	Raisins

Preheat the oven to 400o F.
Core the apples, slice thin, and sprinkle with lemon juice.
Blend Grape Nuts®, pulsing until it's almost pulverized. Spread over the bottom of a covered casserole dish. Dissolve corn starch in 1/3 cup of apple juice and cook until thick.
Mix apples, juice, and spices in a bowl.
Spread the apple mixture over the cereal in the casserole dish.
Sprinkle with additional cinnamon, if desired.
Cover and bake for 45 minutes, or until apples are tender. Remove cover and return to oven to allow pie to brown for 10 to 15 minutes longer. Makes 6 portions.

(1 portion = 127.5 calories, 0.4 grams fat, 5% protein, 93% carbohydrates, 3% fat)

Stovetop Malted Pears

Barley malt gives this dish a sweet yet nutty flavor. You may also dust the pears with spices of your choice. Cinnamon and nutmeg especially lend themselves to fruit-based recipes, but you may prefer to experiment with other flavorings. Be careful, though, until you understand the varieties of taste and how they blend together. Recipes may be as sensitive as chemical formulations, and one false move can spoil the entire dish.

1 can Pear halves (8 oz.), unsweetened and drained, juice reserved

2 Tbsp. Barley Malt sweetener Spices of your choice, ground fine (e.g., cinnamon, nutmeg, cloves)

Open a can of sugar-free pear halves, drain, and move to a dish. Then brush them with microwave-heated barley malt (available at your favorite health food store or specialty food store).

Preheat skillet. Put a touch of the pear juice in the skillet (just enough to keep the malted pears from sticking). Add pears and heat. Serve warm.

Makes 2 portions. (1 portion = 81 calories, 0 gram fat, 1% protein, 99% carbohydrates, 0% fat)

Frozen Desserts

Iced Fruit Cream

4C   Bananas, frozen
¼C   Water or juice

Put 4" segments of frozen bananas pieces in the blender with ¼ cup water or juice. Add more liquid if needed. Blend smooth. Serve immediately.

Makes 8 portions. (1 portion = 111.5 calories, 0.581   grams fat,   4%   protein, 92% carbohydrates, 4% fat)

Top with fresh banana slices, nuts, or cherries. Add other fruits as desired, or no-sugar- added extracts such as strawberries, blueberries, pears, vanilla, maple, and almond.

Strawberry-Banana Pudding

1½ C	Low-fat firm tofu (Mori Nu firm tofu is suggested)
1½ C	Fresh strawberries, sliced
1	Banana
1 tsp.	Vanilla
1 Tbsp.	Lemon juice
¼ tsp.	Salt
2 Tbsp.	Honey

Blend all ingredients together in blender or food processor until creamy and smooth. Pour into individual serving dishes, or pour into individual-sized Grape Nuts® pie shells (make by putting muffin cups in muffin pan then pouring in Grape Nuts®). Chill overnight. Makes 4 to 6 portions. (1 portion = 109.4 calories, 1.886 grams fat, 23% protein, 62% carbohydrates, 15% fat)

Honey Almond Fruit Cocktail

1C	Watermelon
1C	Honeydew melon
1C	Apple
½C	Cantaloupe or pineapple chunks
1	Peach or pear
6 Tbsp.	Agar
2C	Water
1C	Unsweetened soy milk
3 Tbsp.	Honey Almond extract, to taste

Dissolve agar in water, heat.

When completely dissolved, add soy milk, honey, and almond extract, to taste.

Cool and let set. Cut into small chunks.

Cut watermelon, honeydew melon, apple, cantaloupe, and peach or pear into ½" chunks.

Mix agar chunks together with chunks of various fruits for an unusual and colorful fruit cocktail. Makes 8 portions.

(1 portion = 84.72 calories, 0.588 grams fat, 7% protein, 87% carbohydrates, 6% fat)

Haupia

Islanders have enjoyed this local treat for generations. By reducing the quantity of coconut milk, this recipe keeps the fat to a minimum.

2-1/4 C	Rice Dream®
1/4 C	Maple syrup
1/4 C	Coconut milk
2/3 C	Cornstarch
1/2 tsp.	Coconut extract (optional)

Combine 1-1/2 cups Rice Dream® and maple syrup in a saucepan.
Bring to a small boil. Add coconut milk.

Mix together the remaining Rice Dream® and corn-starch in another small bowl. Add to mixture in saucepan, together with coconut extract, mixing constantly until thickened and mixture boils.
Pour into square pan. Cool and cover with plastic wrap. Refrigerate and cut into squares when ready to serve.

Makes 12 portions.

GLYCEMIC INDEX (GI) AND

DR. SHINTANI'S

FOOD MASS INDEX (SMI) TABLES

Glycemic Index. (GI) - Lower is better.

The glycemic index is an index of numbers that represent how high blood sugar will rise in response to the consumption of a specific food. The higher the number, the higher the blood sugar will rise.   It is based on studies of the blood sugar response in normal non-diabetic people when they eat 50 grams of carbohydrate from a specific food. The number is derived by comparing this blood sugar rise to a standard food. The GI(glu) column is a table of numbers comparing blood sugar rise of a food compared to how high blood sugar rises compared to glucose. The GI(bread) column is the blood sugar rise caused by a food compared to how high blood sugar rises compared to white bread. Thus, a food with a lower GI number is preferred.

The Shintani Mass Index (SMI) - Higher is better

The SMI table is the "Shintani Mass Index" which is a table based on the number of pounds required of a specific food to provide one day's worth of calories. It is based on 2500 calories which is an estimated amount of calories for an average man or average active woman. So, for example, the SMI number of apple is 9.6 which means it takes 9.6 pounds of apples to provide 2500 calories or one day's worth of calories. The SMI of boiled potato is 6.4. the SMI value of potato chips is 1.0. This means that it takes 6.4 pounds of boiled potato for a day's worth of calories but only 1 pound of potato chips. You can see that apples or boiled potato will fill your stomach faster than potato chips and you will wind up eating fewer calories if the SMI number is high. An SMI number higher than 4 is considered good because studies show that most people will not eat more than 4.1 pounds of food per day. Thus, a food with a higher SMI number is preferred.

GLYCEMIC INDEX (GI) AND DR.SHINTANI'S FOOD MASS INDEX (SMI)			
Food Item	GI (glu)	GI (bread)	Mass Index
All-Bran®, Kellogg's	42	60	1.4
Angel food cake	67	96	2.1
Apple, dried	29	41	4.6
Apple, fresh	36	51	9.6
Apricot jam	55	79	2.0
Apricots, canned, light syrup	64	91	8.7
Apricots, dried	31	44	4.6
Apricots, fresh	57	81	10.4
Asparagus	*	*	21
Avocado	*	*	3.3
Bacon	*	*	0.8
Bagel, white, frozen	72	103	2.0
Baked beans	48	69	5.1
Banana	53	76	6.0
Banana bread	47	67	1.7
Barley, cracked	50	71	4.5
Barley, pearled	25	36	4.5
Beans, Black	30	43	4.2
Beans, green	*	*	21.9
Beans, Lentils	*	*	5.2
Beans, mung spr	*	*	15.6
Beef, Corned	*	*	1.5
Beef, Ground	*	*	1.9
Beef, steak	*	*	1.2
Beets	64	91	17.8
Black-eyed peas	42	60	5.1
Blueberry Muffin	59	84	2.0
Bran Buds®, Kellogg's	58	83	1.4
Bran Chex®, Nabisco	58	83	1.2
Bran Flakes®, Post	74	106	1.7
Bread stuffing	74	106	2.1
Breadfruit	68	97	4.6

*GI cannot be calculated on some foods because of insufficient carbohydrate in them

GLYCEMIC INDEX (GI) AND DR.SHINTANI'S FOOD MASS INDEX (SMI)			
Food Item	**GI (glu)**	**GI (bread)**	**Mass Index**
BREADS			
Bagel, white, frozen	72	103	2.0
Bread stuffing	74	106	2.1
Bulgur (cracked wheat) bread	58	83	2.2
Corn tortilla	38	54	2.5
Croissant	67	96	1.4
French baguette	95	136	2.0
Hamburger bun	61	87	1.9
Kaiser roll	73	104	1.9
Melba Toast, Old London®	70	100	1.4
Mixed grain bread	45	64	1.9
Oat bran bread	47	67	1.8
Pita bread, white	57	81	2.3
Pumpernickel bread, whole grain	51	73	2.2
Rye bread	65	93	2.4
Rye bread, American light	68	97	1.9
Rye bread, dark	76	109	2.2
Sourdough bread	52	74	2.1
Stone ground whole wheat bread	43	61	2.1
Wheat chapatti	27	39	3.2
White bread	70	100	2.1
Whole wheat bread	69	99	2.2
BREAKFAST CEREALS			
All-Bran®, Kellogg's	42	60	1.4
Bran Buds®, Kellogg's	58	83	1.4
Bran Chex®, Nabisco	58	83	1.2
Bran Flakes®, Post	74	106	1.7
Cheerios®, General Mills	74	106	1.3
Corn Bran®, Quaker	75	107	1.3
Corn Chex®, Nabisco	83	119	1.6
Corn Flakes®, Kellogg's	84	120	1.4

*GI cannot be calculated on some foods because of insufficient carbohydrate in them.

GLYCEMIC INDEX (GI) AND DR.SHINTANI'S FOOD MASS INDEX (SMI)			
Food Item	GI (glu)	GI (bread)	Mass Index
Cream of Wheat®, Instant, Nabisco	74	106	10.3
Cream of Wheat®, Nabisco	66	94	10.7
Golden Grahams®, General Mills	71	101	1.4
grape-nuts®, Post	67	96	1.1
grape-nuts Flakes®, Post	80	114	1.5
Life®, Quaker	66	94	1.4
Muesli, non-toasted	56	80	1.5
Muesli, toasted	43	61	1.5
Nutri-Grain®, Kellogg's	66	94	1.5
Oat Bran Cereal®, Quaker	50	71	1.5
Oat bran, raw	55	79	1.7
Oatmeal (porridge), old-fashioned	59	84	8.9
Oatmeal, one minute instant	66	94	8.9
Puffed Wheat®, Quaker	74	106	1.5
Rice Chex®, General Mills	89	127	1.8
Rice Krispies®, Kellogg's	82	117	1.4
Shredded Wheat®, Nabisco	69	99	1.5
Special K®, Kellogg's	54	77	1.4
Team Flakes®, Nabisco	82	117	1.4
Total®, General Mills	76	109	1.6
Wheat cereal	41	59	9.7
Wheat cereal, quick cooking	54	77	9.1
Broad beans	79	113	7.7
Broccoli	*	*	17.1
Buckwheat	54	77	6.0
Bulgur wheat	48	69	6.6
Bulgur (cracked wheat) bread	58	83	2.2
Butter	*	*	0.8
Butter beans	31	44	6.7
Cabbage	*	*	22.8
Cabbage, Chinese	*	*	39

*GI cannot be calculated on some foods because of insufficient carbohydrate in them.

GLYCEMIC INDEX (GI) AND DR.SHINTANI'S FOOD MASS INDEX (SMI)			
Food Item	GI (glu)	GI (bread)	Mass Index
CAKE			
Angel food cake	67	96	2.1
Banana bread	47	67	1.7
Pound cake	54	77	0.9
Sponge cake	46	66	1.9
CANDY			
Chocolate candy	49	70	1.1
Jelly beans	80	114	2.3
Life Savers®	70	100	1.4
Mars Chocolate Almond Bar®, M&M Mars	68	97	1.2
M&M Chocolate Covered Peanuts®	33	47	1.1
Snickers®, M&M Mars	41	59	1.2
Twix®, Caramel, M&M Mars	44	63	1.1
Cantaloupe	65	93	15.5
Carrots	71	101	12.7
Cashew nuts	*	*	1
Cauliflower	*	*	20.2
Cheerios®, General Mills	74	106	1.3
Cherries	22	31	7.6
Cheese, Cheddar	*	*	1.4
Chicken, dark	*	*	3.1
Chicken, Fried	*	*	2.2
Chicken, white	*	*	3.3
Chocolate candy	49	70	1.1
Collards	*	*	12.1
COOKIES			
Oatmeal cookie	55	79	1.2
Shortbread cookie	64	91	1.1
Social Tea Biscuits®, Nabisco	55	79	1.4
Vanilla wafers	77	110	1.2
Corn	55	79	5.5
Corn Bran®, Quaker	75	107	1.3

*GI cannot be calculated on some foods because of insufficient carbohydrate in them.

GLYCEMIC INDEX (GI) AND DR.SHINTANI'S FOOD MASS INDEX (SMI)			
	GI	GI	Mass
Food Item	(glu)	(bread)	Index
Corn Chex®, Nabisco	83	119	1.6
Corn chips	73	104	1.0
Corn Flakes®, Kellogg's	84	120	1.4
Corn tortilla	38	54	2.5
Cornmeal	68	97	1.5
Couscous	65	93	4.9
Crab	*	*	5.9
Crab Salad	*	*	3.8
CRACKERS			
Graham crackers	74	106	1.4
Rice cakes	82	117	4.4
Rye crispbread, high fiber	65	93	1.4
Soda crackers	72	103	1.3
Stoned wheat thins	67	96	1.5
Wheat Crackers®, Breton	67	96	1.1
Cream cheese	*	*	1.5
Cream of Wheat®, Instant, Nabisco	74	106	10.3
Cream of Wheat®, Nabisco	66	94	10.7
Croissant	67	96	1.4
Cucumbers	*	*	32.8
Dates	103	147	4.0
Doughnut, cake-type	76	109	1.3
Eggplant	*	*	28.8
Eggs	*	*	3.4
Fava beans	79	113	6.9
Fettucini, egg-enriched	32	46	3.9
Fish sticks	38	54	2.0
French baguette	95	136	2.0
French fries	23	33	1.4
Fructose	23	33	1.4

*GI cannot be calculated on some foods because of insufficient carbohydrate in them.

GLYCEMIC INDEX (GI) AND DR.SHINTANI'S FOOD MASS INDEX (SMI)			
Food Item	GI (glu)	GI (bread)	Mass Index
FRUIT AND FRUIT PRODUCTS			
Apple			
Apple, dried	29	41	4.6
Apple, fresh	36	51	9.6
Apricots			
Apricot jam	55	79	2.0
Apricots, canned, light syrup	64	91	8.7
Apricots, dried	31	44	4.6
Apricots, fresh	57	81	10.4
Banana	53	76	6.0
Breadfruit	68	97	4.6
Cantaloupe	65	93	15.5
Cherries	22	31	7.6
Dates	103	147	4.0
Fruit cocktail, canned, light syrup	55	79	17.2
Grapefruit	25	36	18.3
Grapes	43	61	7.7
Kiwi	52	74	9.1
Mango	55	79	8.3
Orange	43	61	11.6
Papaya	58	83	14.3
Peach			
Peach, fresh	28	40	12.8
Peaches, canned, heavy syrup	58	83	7.4
Peaches, canned, light syrup	52	74	10.2
Peaches, canned, natural juice	30	43	12.5
Pear			
Pear, fresh	36	51	9.3
Pears, canned in pear juice, Bartlett	44	63	11.1

*GI cannot be calculated on some foods because of insufficient carbohydrate in them.

GLYCEMIC INDEX (GI) AND DR.SHINTANI'S FOOD MASS INDEX (SMI)			
Food Item	GI (glu)	GI (bread)	Mass Index
Peaches, canned, light syrup	52	74	10.2
Peaches, canned, natural juice	30	43	12.5
Pear			
Pear, fresh	36	51	9.3
Pears, canned in pear juice, Bartlett	44	63	11.1
Pineapple, fresh	66	94	11.1
Plum	24	34	10.1
Raisins	64	91	3.6
Strawberry jam	51	73	2.0
Watermelon	72	103	17.6
Fruit cocktail, canned, light syrup	55	79	17.2
Garbanzo beans, boiled (chickpeas)	33	47	5.2
Garbanzo beans, canned (chickpeas)	42	60	5.6
Glucose	97	139	1.4
Golden Grahams®, General Mills	71	101	1.4
Graham crackers	74	106	1.4
GRAINS			
Barley			
Barley, cracked	50	71	4.5
Barley, pearled	25	36	4.5
Buckwheat	54	77	6.0
Corn			
Corn	55	79	5.5
Corn chips	73	104	1.0
Corn tortilla	38	54	2.5
Cornmeal	68	97	1.5
Popcorn	55	79	1.3
Taco shells, corn	68	97	1.3
Millet	71	101	4.6

*GI cannot be calculated on some foods because of insufficient carbohydrate in them.

GLYCEMIC INDEX (GI) AND DR.SHINTANI'S FOOD MASS INDEX (SMI)			
Food Item	GI (glu)	GI (bread)	Mass Index
Oats			
Oat bran, raw	55	79	1.7
Oatmeal (porridge), old-fashioned	59	84	8.9
Oatmeal, one minute instant	66	94	8.9
Rice			
Rice, brown	55	79	4.9
Rice, instant	91	130	5.6
Rice, specialty (mixed with wild)	55	79	5.4
Rice, white (high amylose)	56	80	5.0
Rice, white, Calrose (low amylose)	83	119	4.6
Rice, white, converted	38	54	4.6
Wheat			
Bulgur wheat	48	69	6.6
Wheat cereal	41	59	9.7
Wheat cereal, quick cooking	54	77	9.1
Wheat chapatti	27	39	3.2
Grapefruit	25	36	18.3
grape-nuts®, Post	67	96	1.1
grape-nuts Flakes®, Post	80	114	1.5
Grapes	43	61	7.7
Hamb, 1/4 lb w ches	*	*	2.1
Hamburger, 1/4 lb	*	*	2.2
Hamburger bun	61	87	1.9
Ham Sandwich	*	*	1.6
Hard Candy	*	*	1.4
Honey	73	104	1.8
Instant noodles, Mr. Noodle®	47	67	4.1
Jelly beans	80	114	2.3
Kaiser roll	73	104	1.9
Kale	*	*	10.3
Kidney beans, boiled	27	39	4.3

*GI cannot be calculated on some foods because of insufficient carbohydrate in them.

GLYCEMIC INDEX (GI) AND DR.SHINTANI'S FOOD MASS INDEX (SMI)			
	GI	GI	Mass
Food Item	(glu)	(bread)	Index
Kidney beans, canned	52	74	6.1
Kiwi	52	74	9.1
Lactose	46	66	1.4
Lentils, green and brown, boiled	29	41	4.7
Life Savers®	70	100	1.4
Life®, Quaker	66	94	1.4
LEGUMES			
Baked beans	48	69	5.1
Black beans	30	43	4.2
Black-eyed peas	42	60	5.1
Broad beans	79	113	7.7
Butter beans	31	44	6.7
Fava beans	79	113	6.9
Garbanzo beans (chickpeas)			
Garbanzo beans, boiled (chickpeas)	33	47	5.2
Garbanzo beans, canned (chickpeas)	42	60	5.6
Kidney beans			
Kidney beans, boiled	27	39	4.3
Kidney beans, canned	52	74	6.1
Lentils, green and brown, boiled	29	41	4.7
Lima beans, baby, frozen	32	46	5.3
Navy (harcort) beans, boiled	38	54	3.9
Pinto beans			
Pinto beans, boiled	39	56	4.0
Pinto beans, canned	45	64	6.2
Soybeans	18	26	3.9
Split peas, yellow and green, boiled	32	46	4.7
Lemon	*	*	30.4
Lettuce	*	*	39
Lima beans, baby, frozen	32	46	5.3
Luncheon Meat	*	*	2.1

*GI cannot be calculated on some foods because of insufficient carbohydrate in them.

GLYCEMIC INDEX (GI) AND DR.SHINTANI'S FOOD MASS INDEX (SMI)			
Food Item	GI (glu)	GI (bread)	Mass Index
Linguini	49	70	3.9
M&M Chocolate Covered Peanuts®	33	47	1.1
Macaroni and cheese, boxed	64	91	3.6
Macaroni, boiled 5 minutes	45	64	3.9
Maltose	105	150	1.4
Mango	55	79	8.3
Margarine	*	*	0.8
Mars Chocolate Almond Bar®, M&M Mars	68	97	1.2
Mayonnaise	*	*	0.8
Melba Toast, Old London®	70	100	1.4
Melon	*	*	18.2
Millet	71	101	4.6
Mixed grain bread	45	64	1.9
Muesli, non-toasted	56	80	1.5
Muesli, toasted	43	61	1.5
Muffin, plain	62	89	1.8
MUFFINS			
Blueberry Muffin	59	84	2.0
Muffin, plain	62	89	1.8
Oat bran muffin	60	86	2.2
Mushrooms	*	*	19.5
Mustard Greens	*	*	17.6
Navy (harcort) beans, boiled	38	54	3.9
Nutri-Grain®, Kellogg's	66	94	1.5
Oat bran bread	47	67	1.8
Oat Bran Cereal®, Quaker	50	71	1.5
Oat bran muffin	60	86	2.2
Oat bran, raw	55	79	1.7
Oatmeal cookie	55	79	1.2
Oatmeal (porridge), old-fashioned	59	84	8.9
Oatmeal, one minute instant	66	94	8.9

*GI cannot be calculated on some foods because of insufficient carbohydrate in them.

GLYCEMIC INDEX (GI) AND DR.SHINTANI'S FOOD MASS INDEX (SMI)			
Food Item	GI (glu)	GI (bread)	Mass Index
Oil/Lard	*	*	0.6
Olives	*	*	4.7
Onions	*	*	14.8
Orange	43	61	11.6
Papaya	58	83	14.3
Parsnips	97	139	6.8
PASTA			
Couscous	65	93	4.9
Fettucini, egg-enriched	32	46	3.9
Instant noodles, Mr. Noodle®	47	67	4.1
Linguini	49	70	3.9
Macaroni and cheese, boxed	64	91	3.6
Macaroni, boiled 5 minutes	45	64	3.9
Ravioli, Duram, meat-filled	39	56	4.4
Spaghetti			
Spaghetti, Duram	55	79	3.7
Spaghetti, white	41	59	3.7
Spaghetti, whole-wheat	37	53	4.4
Tortellini cheese pasta	50	71	3.3
Vermicelli	35	50	3.0
Pastry(danish)	*	*	1.5
Peach, fresh	28	40	12.8
Peaches, canned, heavy syrup	58	83	7.4
Peaches, canned, light syrup	52	74	10.2
Peaches, canned, natural juice	30	43	12.5
Peanuts	14	20	0.9
Pear, fresh	36	51	9.3
Pears, canned in pear juice, Bartlett	44	63	11.1
Peas	48	69	7.0
Pineapple, fresh	66	94	11.1
Pinto beans, boiled	39	56	4.0

*GI cannot be calculated on some foods because of insufficient carbohydrate in them.

GLYCEMIC INDEX (GI) AND DR.SHINTANI'S FOOD MASS INDEX (SMI)			
Food Item	**GI (glu)**	**GI (bread)**	**Mass Index**
Pinto beans, canned	45	64	6.2
Pita bread, white	57	81	2.3
Pizza, cheese	60	86	3.1
Plum	24	34	10.1
Poi	*	*	9.1
Popcorn	55	79	1.3
Potato, baked	85	121	5.9
Potato, boiled, mashed	73	104	6.2
Potato, canned	61	87	9.2
Potato chips	54	77	1.0
Potato, instant	83	119	7.0
Potato, new	62	89	9.1
Potato, sweet	54	77	5.3
Potato, white, baked	60	86	5.9
Potato, white, boiled	56	80	6.4
Potato, white, mashed	70	100	5.2
Potato, white, steamed	65	93	6.4
Pound cake	54	77	0.9
Puffed Wheat®, Quaker	74	106	1.5
Pumpernickel bread, whole grain	51	73	2.2
Pumpkin	75	107	16.3
Radish	*	*	32.1
Raisins	64	91	3.6
Ravioli, Duram, meat-filled	39	56	4.4
Rice, brown	55	79	4.9
Rice cakes	82	117	4.4
Rice Chex®, General Mills	89	127	1.8
Rice, instant	91	130	5.6
Rice Krispies®, Kellogg's	82	117	1.4
Rice, specialty (mixed with wild)	55	79	5.4
Rice, white (high amylose)	56	80	5.0

*GI cannot be calculated on some foods because of insufficient carbohydrate in them.

GLYCEMIC INDEX (GI) AND DR.SHINTANI'S FOOD MASS INDEX (SMI)			
Food Item	GI (glu)	GI (bread)	Mass Index
Rice, white, Calrose (low amylose)	83	119	4.6
Rutabaga	72	103	16.1
Rye bread	65	93	2.4
Rye bread, American light	68	97	1.9
Rye bread, dark	76	109	2.2
Rye crispbread, high fiber	65	93	1.4
Sausages	28	40	1.7
Seaweed(konbu)	*	*	12.7
Seaweed(wakame)	*	*	12.1
Shortbread cookie	64	91	1.1
Shredded Wheat®, Nabisco	69	99	1.5
Shrimp	*	*	4.8
Shrimp, Fried	*	*	2.3
SNACK FOODS			
Corn chips	73	104	1.0
Peanuts	14	20	0.9
Popcorn	55	79	1.3
Potato chips	54	77	1.0
Snickers®, M&M Mars	41	59	1.2
Social Tea Biscuits®, Nabisco	55	79	1.4
Soda crackers	72	103	1.3
Sourdough bread	52	74	2.1
Soybeans	18	26	3.9
Soybean, Sprouts	*	*	11.9
Spaghetti, Duram	55	79	3.7
Spaghetti, white	41	59	3.7
Spaghetti, whole-wheat	37	53	4.4
Special K®, Kellogg's	54	77	1.4
Spinach	*	*	21
Split peas, yellow and green, boiled	32	46	4.7
Sponge cake	46	66	1.9

*GI cannot be calculated on some foods because of insufficient carbohydrate in them.

GLYCEMIC INDEX (GI) AND DR.SHINTANI'S FOOD MASS INDEX (SMI)			
Food Item	**GI (glu)**	**GI (bread)**	**Mass Index**
Squash	*	*	28.8
Stone ground whole wheat bread	43	61	2.1
Stoned wheat thins	67	96	1.5
Strawberry jam	51	73	2.0
Sucrose (table sugar)	65	93	1.4
SUGARS			
Fructose	23	33	1.4
Glucose	97	139	1.4
Honey	73	104	1.8
Lactose	46	66	1.4
Maltose	105	150	1.4
Sucrose (table sugar)	65	93	1.4
Sweet Potato	*	*	5.4
Taco shells, corn	68	97	1.3
Taro	54	77	5.1
Team Flakes®, Nabisco	82	117	1.4
Tofu	*	*	7.6
Tomato	*	*	27.3
Tomato Paste	*	*	6.5
Tortellini cheese pasta	50	71	3.3
Tortilla, corn	59	84	3.0
Tortilla, flour	38	54	2.5
Total®, General Mills	76	109	1.6
Tuna in water	*	*	4.3
Tuna Sandwich	*	*	2.1
Tuna, in oil	*	*	1.9
Turkey	*	*	2.1
Turkey Sandwich	*	*	2.1
Twix®, Caramel, M&M Mars	44	63	1.1
Vanilla wafers	77	110	1.2

*GI cannot be calculated on some foods because of insufficient carbohydrate in them.

GLYCEMIC INDEX (GI) AND DR.SHINTANI'S FOOD MASS INDEX (SMI)			
	GI	GI	Mass
Food Item	(glu)	(bread)	Index
VEGETABLES			
Corn	55	79	5.5
Peas	48	69	7.0
Pumpkin	75	107	16.3
VEGETABLES, ROOT			
Beets	64	91	17.8
Carrots	71	101	12.7
Parsnips	97	139	6.8
Potato			
French fries	75	107	2.5
Potato, baked	85	121	5.9
Potato, boiled, mashed	73	104	6.2
Potato, canned	61	87	9.2
Potato, instant	83	119	7.0
Potato, new	62	89	9.1
Potato, sweet	54	77	5.3
Potato, white, baked	60	86	5.9
Potato, white, boiled	56	80	6.4
Potato, white, mashed	70	100	5.2
Potato, white, steamed	65	93	6.4
Rutabaga	72	103	16.1
Taro	54	77	5.1
Yams	51	73	4.7
Vermicelli	35	50	3.0
Waffles, Aunt Jemima®	76	109	2.8
Watercress	*	*	27.3
Watermelon	72	103	17.6
Wheat cereal	41	59	9.7
Wheat cereal, quick cooking	54	77	9.1
Wheat chapatti	27	39	3.2
Wheat Crackers®, Breton	67	96	1.1

*GI cannot be calculated on some foods because of insufficient carbohydrate in them.

GLYCEMIC INDEX (GI) AND DR.SHINTANI'S FOOD MASS INDEX (SMI)			
Food Item	**GI (glu)**	**GI (bread)**	**Mass Index**
White bread	70	100	2.1
Whole wheat bread	69	99	2.2
Yams	51	73	4.7
Zucchini	*	*	32.1

*GI cannot be calculated on some foods because of insufficient carbohydrate in them.

REFERENCES

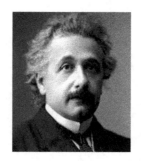

"It is my view that the vegetarian manner of living, by its purely physical effect on the human temperament, would most beneficially influence the lot of mankind"
-Albert Einstein
(1879 - 1955)

PREFACE

[1]Cousens, G. (2005). *Spiritual Nutrition*: North Atlantic Books.

[2]Rosen, S. (1987). *Food for the Spirit*. New York: Bala Books.

[3]Kushi M, Jack A. (1987).*One Peaceful World*. New York, NY. Japan Publications, Inc.

[4]Tuttle, W. (2005). *World Peace Diet*. New York: Lantern Books.

CHAPTER I: Introduction
(No references)

CHAPTER II: Five Lessons for Weight Control, Health, and Peace

[5]Kushi, M. (1996).The book of macrobiotics. New York, NY: Japan Publications, Inc.

[6]Okada, M. (2003) Mokichi okada and health. West Hollywood, CA: Pan American MOA Foundation, Inc.

[7]Steiner, R. (1969) Problems of nutrition. Herndon, VA: Anthroposiphic Press, Inc.

CHAPTER III: Eat More, Weigh Less with the Peace Diet

[8]Shintani, T. (1993). Eat more, weigh less diet. Honolulu, HI: Halpax Publishing.

[9]Poppitt SD, Prentice AM. (1996). Energy density and its role in the control of food intake: evidence from metabolic and community studies. Appetite,26, . 153174.

[10]Shintani, T., Beckham, S., Tang, J., O'Connor, H. K., & Hughes, C. (1999).

[11]Waianae Diet Program: long-term follow-up. Hawaii Medical Journal, 58(5), 117-22.

[12] Tanzi, R. (8/25/2011). Can avoiding meat prevent Alzheimer's? Retrievedfrom . http://www.youtube.com/watch?v=iUaCmTXJWjo.

[13]K T Khaw, N Wareham, S.Bingham, A Welch, R Luben, N Day. (2008). Combined . impact of health behaviours, and mortality in men and women: The EPIC-. Norfolk prospective population study. PLoS Med. 5(1), e12.

CHAPTER IV: Reverse Aging and Disease with the Peace Diet

[14]Singh P, et al. (2003) Does low meat consumption increase life expectancy in . humans? Am J Clin Nutrition, 78(3), 526S-532S.

[15]Merry BJ. (2002). Molecular mechanisms linking calorie restriction and longevity. Int J Biochem & Cell Biology, 34(11), 1340–1354.

[16] M. C. Ruiz, V. Ayala, M. Portero-Otín, J. R. Requena, G. Barja, R. Pamplona. . . (2005). Protein methionine content and MDA-lysine adducts are inversely . related to maximum life span in the heart of mammals. Mechical Ageing . Development 126(10), 1106 - 1114.

[17] M. F. McCarty, J. Barroso-Aranda, F. Contreras. (2009). The low-methionine . content of vegan diets may make methionine restriction feasible as a life . extension strategy. Med. Hypotheses, 72(2), 125-128.

[18] Lazarou J, et al. (1998). Incidence of Adverse Drug Reactions in Hospitalized . Patients. JAMA, 279(15), 1200-1205.

[19] Kaplan, J.R., Clarkson T.B., and Manuck, S.B. (1984). Pathogenesis of carotid . bifurcation atherosclerosis in cynomolgus monkeys, Stroke, 15, 994-1000. Esselstyn, C. B. (2001), Resolving the coronary artery disease epidemic . through plant-based nutrition. Preventive Cardiology, 4, 171–177. doi: . 10.1111/j.1520-037X.2001.00538.x

CHAPTER V: Winning the Cholesterol and Heart Disease Battle

[20] Ornish, D., Brown, S. E., Scherwitz, L. W., Billings, J. H., Armstrong, W. T., Ports, T. A., et al. (1990). Can lifestyle changes reverse coronary heart disease? . The lifestyle heart trial. Lancet, 336(8708), 129-33.

[21] Brody, J. (1990, May 8). Huge Study of Diet Indicts Fat and Meat. The New York . Times. Retrieved from . http://www.nytimes.com/1990/05/08/science/huge-study-of-diet-indicts-. fat-and-meat.html?src=pm&pagewanted=1.

[22] Campbell, T.C. (2005). The China Study. Dallas,TX: Benabella Books.

[23] John A. McDougall, J.A., McDougall, M. (2014). Dr. McDougall's Health and . Medical Center. Retrieved from http://www.drmcdougall.com/about/dr-. john-mcdougall/.

[24] Esselstyn, C.B., Jr. (2007). Prevent and reverse heart disease. New York, NY: Avery.

[25] Ornish, D., Brown, S. E., Scherwitz, L. W., Billings, J. H., Armstrong, . W. T., Ports, T. A., et al. (1990). Can lifestyle changes reverse coronary .heart disease? The Lifestyle Heart Trial. Lancet, 336(8708), 129-33.

[26] Campbell, T. C. (2005). The China study. Dallas, TX: Benabella Books. Slutsker L., Hoesly F.C., Miller L., Williams L.P., Watson J.C., Fleming . D.W. (1990).

[27] Eosinophilia-myalgia syndrome associated with exposure to tryptophan from a

CHAPTER VI: Bringing Peace to the Inflammation in Your Body
single .   manufacturer. JAMA 264(2), 213–7.

[28] Dean, A. & Armstrong, J. (5/8/2009). Genetically modified foods. American . Academy of Environmental Medicine. Retrieved from . http://www.aaemonline.org/gmopost.html

[29] Esposito, K. et al. (2002). Inflammatory cytokine concentrations are acutely increased by hyperglycemia in humans. Circulation,106, 2067-2072.

CHAPTER VII: Control Blood Sugar and Diabetes with a Carbohydrate Revolution

[30]Pihlajaaki J. et al. (2004). Insulin resistance is associated with increased cholesterol . synthesis and decreased cholesterol absorption in normoglycemic men. J . Lipid Res., Mar;45(3), 507-12. Epub 2003 Dec 1.

[31]Ginsberg H.N. (2000). Insulin resistance and cardiovascular disease. J Clin . Invest.,106, 453-458.

CHAPTER VIII: The Peace Diet and Cancer

[32]Campbell, T. C. (2005). The China Study. Dallas, TX: Benabella Books.

[33]High dose vitamin C. (2013/5/28). CNN. Retrieved from . http://www.cancer.gov/cancertopics/pdq/cam/highdosevitaminc/

[34]Lappe, J.M. et al. (2007). Vitamin D and calcium supplementation reduces cancer . risk: Results of a randomized trial. Am J Clin Nutr., 85, 1586-91. `

[35]Cavuoto P., Fenech, M.F. (2012) A review of methionine dependency and the role of .methionine restriction in cancer growth control and life-span extension. Cancer Treat. Rev., 38(6), 726-736.

[36]Fawcett, A. & Smith, C. (1992). Cancer Free: 30 Who Triumphed Over Cancer . Naturally: Japan:Japan Publications.

CHAPTER IX: The Physiology of Peace

[37]Beezhold, B. L. & Johnston, C. S. (2012). Restriction of meat, fish, and poultry in . omnivores improves mood: A pilot randomized controlled trial. Nutrition . Journal, 11:9.

[37]Beezhold, B. L., Johnston, C. S., Daigle, D. R. (2010). Vegetarian diets are . associated with healthy mood states: A cross-sectional study in seventh day Adventist adults. Nutr J, 9, 26.

[38]Dorgan, J., Judd, J., Longcope, C., Brown, C., Schatzkin, A., Clevidence, B., et al. . .(1996). Effects of dietary fat and fiber on plasma and urine androgens and estrogens in men: a controlled feeding study. The American Journal of . Clinical Nutrition, 64(6), 850-5.

[39]Dorgan, J., Judd J. T., Longcope C., Brown C., Schatzkin A., Clevidence B.A., . Campbell W.S., Nair P.P., Franz C., Kahle L., Taylor, P.R. (1996). Effects . of dietary fat and fiber on plasma and urine androgens and estrogens in . men: a controlled feeding study. Am J Clin Nutr., 64(6), 850-5.

[40]Hayes T.B., Collins A., Lee M., et al. (2002). Hermaphroditic, demasculinized frogs after exposure to the herbicide atrazine at low ecologically relevant doses. . Proc. Natl. Acad. Sci. U.S.A., 99(8), 5476–80.

[41]Genetically modified foods. (5/8/2009). American Academy of Environmental . Medicine. Retreived from http://www.aaemonline.org/gmopost.html

[42]Fergusona, D.M., Warner, R.D. (2008). Have we underestimated the impact of pre-slaughter stress on meat quality in ruminants?). Meat Science 80, 12–. 19. Retrieved from http://www.scn.org/~bk269/fear.html/

[43]Wurtman, R. J. and Wurtman, J. J. (1995), Brain serotonin, carbohydrate-craving, . obesity and depression. Obesity Research, 3, 477S–480S. 6 SEP 2012 DOI: 10.1002/j.1550-8528.1995.tb00215.x

[44]Beezhold B.L., Johnston C.S., Daigle D.R. (2009). Preliminary evidence that . vegetarian diet improves mood. American Public Health Association annual conference, November 7-11, 2009. Philadelphia, PA.

[45]Esposito G, Giovacchini et al. (2008). Imaging neuroinflammation in Alzheimer's . disease with radiolabeled arachidonic acid and PET. J Nucl Med. 49(9), . 1414-21.

[46]Tanzi, R. (2011, Aug 25). Can avoiding meat prevent Alzheimer's? Retrieved from http://www.youtube.com/watch?v=iUaCmTXJWjo

CHAPTER X: ANATOMY OF PEACE
(No references)

CHAPTER XI: The Peace Diet: More than Karma Free
[47]Luna, a wild orca boy, tries to communicate with humans by imitating their boat's . motor. Wimp.com. Retrieved from . http://www.wimp.com/communicatehumans/

[48]Warrick J. (2001, April 11). Modern meat: A brutal harvest. They die piece by piece. Washington Post, April 11, 2001.

[49]Robbins J. (1987). Diet for a New America. Novato, California: New World Library.

[50]Cassidy, E., West, P., Gerber, J., & Foley, J. (2013). Redefining agricultural yields: . from tonnes to people nourished per hectare. Environmental Research . Letters, 8:034015.

CHAPTER XII: Ancient Wisdom for Modern Health and Peace
[51]Holy Bible: New International Version. (2011). Grand Rapids, Mich.: Zondervan.
[52]Holy Bible: New International Version. (2011). Grand Rapids, Mich.: Zondervan.
[53]Holy Bible: New International Version. (2011). Grand Rapids, Mich.: Zondervan.
[54]Szekely, E. B. (1981). Essene Gospel of Peace. London: International Biogenic Society.
[55]Rosen, S. (1987). Food for the Spirit. New York: Bala Books, 36.
[56]Rosen, S. (1987). Food for the Spirit. New York: Bala Books, 26.
[57]Chrysostom, Saint John. (2014). All-Creatures.org. Retrieved from http://www.all-creatures.org/quotes/chrysostom_john.html.
[58]Paul, T. (2000). Hinduism and Vegetarianism. International Vegetarian Union. . Retrieved from http://www.ivu.org/news/march2000/hinduism.html.
[59]Ancient India and The East: Zoroaster. (2010, April 6). International Vegetarian Union. Retrieved from http://www.ivu.org/history/east/zoroaster.html.
[60]Khalsa, S. K. K. (2010). Sikh spiritual practice. Needs city, UK: John Hunt . Publishing Ltd.
[61]Shah, B. S. (2002). Introduction to jainism: Needs city and state. Setubandh . Publications.

[62]Warren, H. C. (2005). Buddhism in translations: Needs city and state. Harvard University Press.de Bary, W. T., et al. (1958). Sources of indian tradition. New York: .Columbia University Press.

[63]Suzuki, D. (1932). The lankavatara sutra. London: Routledge.

[64]Cousens, G. (2000). Conscious eating. Berkeley, Calif: North Atantic Books.

[65]Hai, C. (need year). The key of immediate enlightenment. Taipei, Formosa: The . Supreme Master Ching Hai International Association Publishing Co., Ltd.

[66]Kapleau, P., Kapleau, R. P. (1986). To cherish all life: A buddhist case for becoming vegetarian. Need city, state: publisher.

[67]Fujii, M. (2005). The enlightened kitchen. Tokyo, Japan: Kodansha International, . Ltd.

CHAPTER XIII: Dr. Shintani's Peace Diet Plate

[68]Fruits and Vegetables. (2013, September 12). Centers for Disease Control and . Prevention. Retrieved . from:http://www.cdc.gov/nutrition/everyone/fruitsvegetables/index.html

[69]Marsh, AG; et al. (1988). Vegetarian lifestyle and bone mineral density. Am J C, 48, 837-41.

[70]Richards, Graham. (1987). Human evolution. London, England: Routledge and . Kegan Paul.

[71]Deopurkar R., Ghanim H., Friedman J., Abuaysheh S., Sia C. L., Mohanty P., . Viswanathan P., Chaudhuri A., Dandona P. (2010, May). Differential effects of cream, glucose, and orange juice on inflammation, endotoxin, and the . expression of Toll-like receptor-4 and suppressor of cytokine signaling-3. . Diabetes Care, 2010 May; 33(5), 991-7.

[72]Mansueto,P., A Seidita, D'Alcamo,A., Carroccio, A. Non-celiac gluten sensitivity: . Literature review. J Am Coll Nutr 2014 33(1), 39–54.

[73]Darmadi-Blackberry, I., Wahlqvist, M., Kouris-Blazos,A., et al. (2004). Legumes: . the most important dietary predictor of survival in older people of different ethnicities. Asia Pac J Clin Nutr. 13(2), 217-20.

[74]Bouchenak, M., Lamri-Senhadji, M. (2013).Nutritional quality of legumes, and their role in cardiometabolic risk prevention: A review. J Med Food, 16(3), 185 – 198.

[75]Singhal P., Kaushik, G., Mathur, P. (2013). Antidiabetic potential of commonly . consumed legumes: A review. Crit Rev Food Sci Nutr., 54(5), 655 – 672.

CHAPTER XIV: The Whole Person Peace Diet Plan

[76]Steiner, R. (1997). The effects of esoteric development. The Hague, Netherlands: . Anthroposophic Books.

[77]Position Paper on GMO Foods, American Academy of Environmental Medicine. . This needs more information – author, year, title.

[78]The Showa Denko Tryptophan disaster reevaluated. (6/9/2013). Physicians and . Scientists for Responsible Application of Science and Technology Retrived from http://www.psrast.org/demsd.htm.

[79]Kutlu A., Oztürk S., Taşkapan O., Onem Y., Kiralp M.Z., Ozçakar L. (2010). Meat-induced joint attacks, or meat attacks the joint: rheumatism versus allergy. . Nutr. Clin. Practice, Feb; 25(1), 90-1.

[80]Carrasco-Gallardo C., Guzmán L., Maccioni R.B. (2012). Shilajit: A natural . phytocomplex with potential procognitive activity. Int J Alzheimers Dis. . 2012, 674142.

[81]Unlock the secret of longevity. (4/1/2010). Retrieved from . http://shifuyanlei.blogspot.com/2010/04/unlock-secret-of-longevity.html

[82]Apau- Ludlum, N., Shintani, T., Harrigan, R. (2012) Scalar field therapy and . mitigation of seizure disorder: A case report. J Neurol Res. 2 (4), 172-175

[83]Mills E, et al. (2005). Melatonin in the treatment of cancer: A systematic review of . randomized controlled trials and meta-analysis. Journal of Pineal Research, 2005,39(4), 360-366.

[84]Anderson J. W., Liu C., Kryscio R. J. (2008) Blood pressure response to . transcendental meditation: a meta-analysis. American Journal of . Hypertension, 21(3), 310-316.

[85]Emmons, R. A., & McCullough, M. E. (2003). Counting blessings versus burdens: . An experimental investigation of gratitude and subjective well-being in daily life. Journal of Personality and Social Psychology, 84(2), 377-89.

[86]Sansone, R. A., & Sansone, L. A. (2010). Gratitude and well being: The benefits of . appreciation. Psychiatry, 7(11), 18-22.

[87]Grant, A. M., & Gino, F. (2010). A little thanks goes a long way: Explaining why . gratitude expressions motivate prosocial behavior. Journal of Personality . and Social Psychology, 98(6), 946-55.

[88]Lambert, N. M., & Fincham, F. D. (2011). Expressing gratitude to a partner leads . to more relationship maintenance behavior. Emotion, 11(1), 52-60.

CPSIA information can be obtained
at www.ICGtesting.com
Printed in the USA
LVHW061501170723
752631LV00027B/226